CNOR® Exam Study Guide

3rd Edition

Produced by CCI, the
official governing body of the
CNOR® certification program.

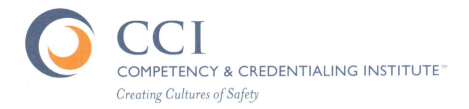

CCI
COMPETENCY & CREDENTIALING INSTITUTE™
Creating Cultures of Safety

Published by
Competency & Credentialing Institute
2170 South Parker Road, Suite 295
Denver, CO 80231

CNOR® Exam Study Guide

3rd Edition

Produced by CCI, the official governing body of the CNOR certification program.

This preparation guide has been developed to provide resources and guidance for the perioperative nurse who is preparing for the CNOR examination. The perioperative nurse's scope of practice has been used as the overall basis for the organization of this publication and also serves as the basic framework for each chapter.

The Competency & Credentialing Institute presents this publication to enhance the knowledge and skill level of the perioperative nurse who strives to demonstrate achievement in practice. Using this book as a study guide, however, is not required, nor does it guarantee successfully passing the exam.

Printed in the United States of America

978-0-9884315-5-3   CNOR Exam Study Guide, Third Edition (2014)

Table of Contents

Chapter 4   Communication 143

Chapter 5   Transfer of Care 159

Chapter 6   Cleaning, Disinfecting, Packaging, Sterilizing, Transporting, and Storing Instruments and Supplies............. 175

PREFACE

Julie Mower, MSN, RN, CNS, CNOR
Credentialing and Education Project Manager
Competency & Credentialing Institute

Earning the CNOR® credential is a highly sought after professional and personal goal. As a certified perioperative nurse, you demonstrate your competency every day in support of quality patient care. CCI wants to help you achieve this professional milestone by providing materials to help you prepare for your certification exam.

The *CNOR Exam Study Guide* is just one of many tools that CCI offers as an aid to your preparation for the CNOR examination. Depending on your level of experience, it may be necessary to access other resources in addition to this book, because the CNOR exam is a comprehensive assessment of every facet of perioperative nursing practice.

This *Guide* is designed to build on your current knowledge and experience by providing opportunities to engage in critical-thinking exercises. Interactive learning activities ask you to apply current best practices to common clinical situations encountered by a nurse with two years of experience. It is highly recommended that you use the references cited in each module to complete the exercises in this book. The answers to the questions on the CNOR exam are based on these same references.

Before you start reviewing the material, please note that this *Guide* contains features that help to make it a more useful preparation tool. These include:

- A section titled "How To Use This Book" that outlines the book format and learning activities (page 11).

- A section titled "Strategies for Success: Getting Prepared and Being Test-Wise" to help you prepare to take the exam. You will find information on the process involved in answering multiple-choice questions and test-taking strategies from an exam development expert (page 16).

- A self-assessment to help you evaluate your current knowledge and skills and guide you in developing your own study plan (page 29).

- A learning needs assessment that matches current knowledge with content on the exam (page 31).

- A study plan with a suggested template for organizing and focusing on key components of the exam (Appendix A, pages 269-279).

- A list of the domains covered in the exam, with pertinent topics listed under each domain to help guide your studying (Appendix B, pages 280-286).

- CCI online resources, including more than 50 of CCI's popular "Questions of the Week" with detailed answers and extensive references; concept map templates; test and study resources; learning needs and self-assessment forms; and test prep webinars. Go to the Study Guide Toolbox at http://www.cc-institute.org/toolbox

Studies show that people retain more information when they use an interactive learning approach that includes reading the information, talking about it, and writing it. We encourage you to use this workbook as the basis for studying with a group of your peers and fellow exam-takers. You may also want to contact a CCI Champion in your institution for guidance. CCI Champions understand the value of certification and help mentor nurses seeking the CNOR credential. A list of Champions is available on our web site (www.cc-institute.org) under the "Champions" tab.

If you have questions about this *Guide* or preparing for the CNOR exam, please contact CCI at (888) 257-2667. ***Good luck as you embark on this exciting phase of your career.***

Developmental Editor

Terri Goodman, PhD, RN, CNOR
Consultant
Terri Goodman and Associates
Dallas, Texas

Contributing Authors

Victoria Dreger, MSN, MA, RN, CNOR, CNL
Nurse Clinician III
Advocate Christ Medical Center
Oak Lawn, Illinois

Peter Graves, BSN, RN, CNOR
Surgical Services Manager
Baylor Medical Center
Carrollton, Texas

Ramie Miller, BSN, RN, CNOR
Staff Nurse
Ochsner-Baptist Medical Center
New Orleans, Louisiana

Julie Mower, MSN, RN, CNS, CNOR
Project Manager
Competency & Credentialing Institute
Denver, Colorado

April Sappe, BSN, BS, RN, CNOR
Staff Nurse
Miami Valley Hospital
Dayton, Ohio

Hope Shaw, MSN, BA, RN, CNOR
Faculty
Southeastern College
Miami Lakes, Florida

Teresa K. Velez, MSN, ARNP, NP-C, CRNFA, CNOR, ONC
ARNP Surgical First Assistant
Florida Hospital Memorial Medical Center
Daytona Beach, Florida

Linda D. Waters, PhD, RN
Vice President
Prometric
Baltimore, Maryland

Reviewers

Ruth Aughe, BSN, RN, CNOR, CRNFA
Clinical Nursing Educator
Montgomery County Memorial Hospital
Red Oak, Iowa

Peggy Brewer, MSN, RN, CNOR
Staff Nurse, Operating Room
Soliant Health Care
Tucker, Georgia

Ann C. From, MS, RN, CNOR
Nursing Clinical Educator, Perioperative Services
Ben Taub General Hospital
Houston, Texas

Gail Horvath, MSN, RN, CNOR, CRCST
Patient Safety Analyst/Consultant
ECRI Institute
Plymouth Meeting, Pennsylvania

Christopher Peredney, MSN, MS, RN, CNOR
Assistant Clinicial Manager/Interim Manager, Main OR
Franciscan Health Services, St. Joseph's Medical Center
Tacoma, Washington

Patricia Seifert, MSN, RN, CNOR, CRNFA, FAAN
Staff Nurse/RN First Assistant/Educator
Inova Heart and Vascular Institute
Falls Church, Virginia

Kim Wheeler, MSN, RN, CNOR
Interim Nurse Manager, Operating Room
Lahey Hospital and Medical Center
Burlington, Massachusetts

Graphics

Masako James
Aurora, Colorado

Note: Concept maps created with templates from https://bubbl.us.

INTRODUCTION

How To Use This Book

Overview

This book is probably different from other study guides you may have used to prepare for exams. It certainly is different from previous *Guides to CNOR Exam Preparation*. Instead of providing a summary of a specific topic with sample test questions, the format has been reversed — you are expected to bring the knowledge accrued from your years of experience and your readings of recommended reference materials, and apply it to problem-based scenarios and questions that are based on actual clinical situations. These learning activities should not be considered all-inclusive for what will be covered on the exam; rather, they should be viewed as "brain templates," or a way to approach problem-solving any clinical issue. It is hoped that this active thinking process will serve you well, not only for the purposes of studying for the exam, but also in your professional practice. After all, passing the exam is just the beginning, not the end, of your continued quest for competence.

Getting Ready: References and Resources

Hypothetically, if one has experience with a variety of types of cases in a work environment that supports current best practices, it may not be necessary to study for the exam at all. Your practice would already mirror the correct answers on the exam. However, most of us feel more secure reviewing the topics that will be covered on the exam. It's important to remember that the exam is based on best practices as reflected in the current literature, which may differ from the clinical practice at any one facility.

Although there are many quality perioperative resources available on the market today, both this *Guide* and the exam are based on information found in three key reference books. Use the most current edition of each of these books for studying. Best practices change over time (how many of us remember doing a pre-op shave for our patient the night before surgery?), and you will not save money by purchasing or borrowing outdated materials and possibly jeopardizing your chances of successfully passing the exam.

Reading assignments from these books are included at the beginning of each module in this guide. Using these books will help you respond to the learning activities and prepare for the content covered on the exam.

Required Reference

• AORN. (2014). *Perioperative Standards and Recommended Practices*. Denver.

This is the primary resource that guides our perioperative practice. It may be purchased at www.aorn.org. Being a member of AORN allows you to purchase this book, as well as other references in their bookstore, at a discount. Members also receive a discount on the CNOR exam application fee. Supporting AORN is an important part of our responsibility as professional perioperative nurses. Along with the CNOR credential, it demonstrates a commitment to quality, safe patient care.

Highly Recommended References

Either of the following will be sufficient; it is not necessary to purchase both of them.

• Phillips, N. (ed.). (2013). *Berry and Kohn's Operating Room Technique*. St. Louis: Mosby.

• Rothrock, J. (ed.). (2015). *Alexander's Care of the Patient in Surgery*. St. Louis: Mosby.

Depending on your clinical practice, you may want to supplement these books with additional resources on pharmacology, pathophysiology, or diagnostic/lab values. Space prevents a more extensive list, but a sampling of recently published books is provided below. This list is not all-inclusive, and there are many other good references available. It's important to find a book that is easy for you to use and that contains the most current information available.

Tip for Success

Before going through the expense of purchasing any of these books, see if you can borrow references from your facility library, unit manager, perioperative educator, or other staff members who may either have recently taken the exam or are in the process of studying.

Pathophysiology

• McCance, K.L., Huether, S.E. (2010). *Pathophysiology: The Biologic Basis for Disease in Adults and Children*. Maryland Heights, MO: Mosby Elsevier.

• Porth, C. (2014). *Essentials of Pathophysiology: Concepts of Altered Health States*. Philadelphia, PA: Wolters Kluwer Health/Lippincott Williams and Wilkin.

Laboratory/Diagnostic Tests

- Kee, J. L. (2013). *Laboratory and Diagnostic Tests with Nursing Implications.* Upper Saddle River, NJ: Prentice Hall.

- Pagana, K.D. & Pagana, T.J. (2013). *Mosby's Manual of Diagnostic and Laboratory Tests.* St. Louis: Mosby Elsevier.

Pharmacology

- Vallerand, A., & Sanoski, C. (2013). *Davis' Drug Guide for Nurses*. Philadelphia: F.A. Davis.

- Lacy, C.F., Armstrong, L.L., Goldman, M.P., & Lance, L.L. (eds.). *Drug Information Handbook 2013-2014: A Comprehensive Resource for All Clinicians and Healthcare Professionals.* Philadelphia: Lexicomp, Inc./Wolters Kluwer Health.

Nursing Diagnoses

- AORN. (2011). *Perioperative Nursing Data Set.* Denver.

> ## Tip for Success
>
> Your facility may already have an online formulary available for you to use at no cost. An excellent online resource is epocrates (https://online.epocrates.com/home). It's free, is updated frequently, and can be downloaded to your PDA or smart phone.

Making This Guide Work for You

Each chapter in this guide is based on a domain, or topic, found on the exam. The format of this book encourages you to write in it, reflect on your progress, and identify your strengths and areas for improvement. Make it your own. Each chapter is organized as follows.

The *percentage of questions* on a particular domain is found at the beginning of the chapter. If study time is in short supply, this may help you organize your time by focusing on the chapters with the highest percentage of questions.

Modules are organized based on the tasks and knowledge statements found in each domain (see Appendix B). They help organize the "chunks" of information and make the process of studying more manageable.

Competency outcomes are provided for successfully completing the chapter. This allows you to quickly check to see if you already know the content, or will need to review it.

Detailed *reading assignments* cover the content for the domain. This information will also be used to complete the learning activities.

Key words help to further focus your reading on relevant content.

Case study activities are based on our sample patient, introduced in Chapter 1.

Learning activities require application of the content from the reading assignments and prerequisite knowledge and skills. These learning activities may be any combination of short answer, fill in the blank, multiple choice, or scenario-based.

Skill building activities encourage you to take advantage of additional learning opportunities in your clinical setting.

The *summary* at the end of each chapter provides "golden rules" for competent practice.

A *glossary* at the end of each chapter defines words or terms that may be unfamiliar.

Answers to learning activities are provided at the end of each chapter.

Additional *readings and resources* are included at the end of each module.

How to Use Online Resources

Supplemental information, found at http://www.cc-institute.org/toolbox, may be used to enhance the activities in the *Study Guide*. Clinical questions that encourage dialogue with your peers and critical thinking and links to CCI website materials ensure that you are getting the most up-to-date information on perioperative issues.

A Note on Taking Practice Tests

Many people like to use sample tests as part of their studying routine. This is in no way a requirement for successfully passing the exam. If you decide to purchase practice questions, the following information will be helpful in maximizing their usefulness.

The purposes of the sample test questions are twofold: to provide an experience similar to taking the actual CNOR exam, and to evaluate your knowledge of a particular topic. These multiple-choice questions are comparable in form and content to the types of questions on the actual CNOR certification exam. If testing anxiety is a concern, completing the practice test should mirror the actual exam as closely as possible. Resist the urge to immediately look up the answer to each question. You won't be able to do this on the actual exam, which may be a source of additional anxiety on testing day.

Many nurses find answering practice test questions helpful in preparing for the exam, but it is important to understand this tool's limitations. First, these questions WILL NOT be found on the actual exam. The practice questions should not be used as a substitute for studying. Answering the sample questions multiple times has limited benefit, as you will begin to memorize not only the answers, but the questions, which diminishes their value as a tool to evaluate what you know or don't know. Other tips for utilizing the practice questions to their fullest potential:

- For all the questions, look up the rationale in your text books, whether you answered the question correctly or not. Active involvement in the learning process means you'll be more likely to remember the content, and provides the "why" that you can then apply to similar questions.

- Look at trends; missing multiple questions in a single domain (for example, preoperative assessment or emergency situations) means extra studying and/or clinical exposure is needed in those areas.

- Take the "big picture" view of incorrect answers; missing a question on a particular drug means you will want to review that drug, but it may also signify a knowledge deficit in pharmacology in general.

It is important to remember that the level of success in answering the practice questions in no way transfers to success on the actual exam. More preparation ideas for test-taking can be found in CCI's *CNOR Candidate Handbook* (www.cc-institute.org) and in the next section.

Guide to Activities

Several types of activities are included in this *Guide*. Activities to be completed within the printed book include matching, fill-in-the-blank, and other types of exercises. An example of a matching activity is shown at the right.

Activities that require the learner to seek outside information or perform tasks outside the printed book (e.g., online) are called "Go To" Activities and appear in a framed box.

Exercises related to the Case Study introduced in Chapter One are labeled as such and outlined in orange.

Activity — Matching
EXAMPLE: From the list of patient assessment data below, write . . .

"Go To" Activity
EXAMPLE: Go to Question of the Week # 6, NPO Status, in the Study Guide Toolbox at http://www.cc-institute.org/toolbox . . .

Case Study Activity
EXAMPLE: How does Mr. J.'s allergy to shellfish affect . . .

Let's Get Started!

By now you are either excited about starting on your journey to validate your practice as a competent perioperative nurse, or are overwhelmed at the magnitude of the task ahead. Both emotions are totally normal. Just remember that the test is based on what a nurse with two years of practice is expected to know. As a person eligible to take the exam, you already have met this criterion. So... let's get started!

Strategies for Success: Getting Prepared and Being Test-Wise

Contributing author: Linda D. Waters, PhD, RN

Being successful at passing the CNOR certification examination for perioperative nursing requires having a thorough and sound foundation of the knowledge and skills required for competent clinical practice, as well as an understanding of the test-taking process. Knowledge is attained through work experiences and independent learning, as well as through formal educational programs. The experiential component requires that an individual who is eligible to take the CNOR certification examination has a minimum of two years of work experience in perioperative nursing. The knowledge component is acquired through a variety of learning activities, including formal education, self-study, and continuing education programs, all aiming to promote continuing competency. It is the combination of experiential and cognitive knowledge that forms the foundation of expert clinical practice.

In addition to evidence-based clinical knowledge, you will also need to have a firm understanding of the testing process. Being familiar with the testing process will not only prepare you to take the test and enable you to feel more confident about the testing experience, but will also acquaint you with the environment in which the test will be given. There is a definite skill in answering multiple-choice test questions. Becoming familiar with techniques for responding to multiple-choice questions will improve your chances of successful performance on the CNOR certification examination.

This chapter provides information about planning your personalized study program, obtaining the necessary resources to assist in your preparation, understanding the processes involved in answering multiple-choice test questions, and developing sound test-taking strategies to lead to success on your CNOR certification examination.

Learning Objectives

Upon completion of this section, the individual will be able to:

1. Identify specific content areas in perioperative nursing where further study is needed.
2. Develop an action plan and timeline for acquiring additional knowledge in content areas where needed.
3. Identify resources that will be of assistance in preparing for the CNOR certification examination.
4. Identify the major features of multiple-choice test questions.
5. Develop skill in applying test-taking strategies when answering multiple-choice test questions.

Developing Good Study Habits

Making the initial commitment to take a certification examination is an important decision. For most test takers, becoming certified in a specialty area of nursing practice accomplishes both personal and professional goals. The personal goal is a feeling of accomplishment — tackling a task that may be difficult yet, at the same time, rewarding. Professionally, certification provides external recognition of excellence in nursing and may promote career advancement. In addition, certification is a symbol of achievement that distinguishes the credential holder from others in the field. The certification holder can proudly state that he or she has met a high standard of achievement established by experts in perioperative nursing. It is truly an accomplishment to acquire certification as a CNOR.

An important step in the certification process is determining what your personal investment will be in preparing for the examination. And what a personal investment it is! Perhaps the easiest actions are completing the application and paying the examination fee. The more difficult part is realistically determining what you need to do and can do to prepare for the examination. Each person will need to decide what works best for him or her. Ultimately, when you go to take your examination, you want to be certain you are as prepared as you can be and are confident about your ability to demonstrate your command of perioperative nursing knowledge.

Preparing to take the CNOR examination may seem like an overwhelming task. Answering the following questions may help organize your study plan.

Question #1 — Should I study for the examination?

Studying for the examination is your choice and is, in no small way, a decision based on your years of experience in perioperative nursing. While experience is critical, your personal work experiences may not have provided you with the broad range of skills and knowledge needed to be successful on the certification examination. Remember, a certification examination is a general examination that will ask questions about many areas of perioperative nursing. Ask yourself whether your experiences in perioperative nursing have been broad enough to prepare you for all content areas that might be included on the test. Are there areas of practice with which you have not had work experience or where standards of practice may have recently changed?

So, do you need to study? Conduct a self-assessment to determine your chances for passing the certification examination. How do you do that?

An excellent starting point is to review critical documents, including the *CNOR Candidate Handbook*, found at www.cc-institute.org; the CNOR Exam Study Plan; and the current AORN *Perioperative Standards and Recommended Practices*. Turn to page 31 to complete your learning needs assessment. Assess your "level of competency" for each content area. Conduct this assessment before you register and schedule your examination to allow sufficient preparation time before the examination. Use a rating scale such as the one below to determine what you believe to be your current level of competency.

1 — Very Certain: I know this content area well and believe that my work experiences have fully prepared me. I am comfortable with current practices and believe I am up-to-date with new developments and advances.

2 — Certain: I am reasonably comfortable with this content area and believe that my work experiences have prepared me fairly well.

3 — Undecided: I have some knowledge and some experiences in this area, but there may be a few content areas where I am not as strong or for which my work experiences have not fully prepared me. I may not be current in all areas of perioperative nursing.

4 — Uncertain: I am aware that I have some knowledge deficits and/or a lack of work experience in this content area. I will need to engage in some study or other remediation to be comfortable with this content area.

5 — Very Uncertain: I am aware that I have many knowledge deficits and/or lack work experiences in this content area. These areas of weakness will require me to engage in remediation activities before taking the examination.

Apply this rating scale to each domain of the *CNOR Candidate Handbook*. Be completely honest with your learning assessment — remember, it is intended to help you prepare for the CNOR examination. If you rate all areas as 1 or 2, you may find that you will need little to no preparation before taking the examination. If, on the other hand, you find that you have a mixture of responses, rating some content areas 1 and 2 and others 3, 4, or 5, you may find it very useful to develop an individualized study plan that will allow you sufficient time to prepare before taking the examination. Appendix B (pages 280-286) has a more detailed breakdown of subjects included in each section, or domain, of the exam.

Knowing that you have done all you can to prepare for taking the CNOR certification examination will give you that extra boost of confidence and reduce anxiety! It also will help you determine when to schedule your examination within the testing window.

Be realistic! Preparing for the examination will be best completed over a period of weeks, not days or hours. Unexpected events will occur which may take away from your preparation time. Don't shortchange yourself. Allow sufficient study time before the examination.

Question #2 — What is the most important content to study?

Go back to the learning needs assessment you completed when making the decision whether to study. Consider dividing the content areas from the *CNOR Candidate Handbook* into three broad areas:

Area 1 — Content that I have knowledge strengths.

Area 2 — Content that is mixed; I may know some areas but have weaknesses in others.

Area 3 — Content that I know I have knowledge weaknesses.

Then look at the proportion of the test that is dedicated to each area you identified (Appendix C, page 287). Concentrate your study time on those areas where you have the greatest knowledge weaknesses and where the largest percentage of test questions will be represented. Tackle those needs FIRST, before going on to other areas. Each chapter in this study guide outlines the percentage of questions found on that topic on the examination.

Question #3 — What is the best study style for me?

Once you have decided that you do want to study for the examination and you have developed a study plan specific to your needs, next determine a study style that works best for you. Remember back to your school days. What worked best for you then? Were you more successful when you studied alone in the privacy of your own study space? Or were you more focused when you studied with others? Maybe a combination study style works best for you — individual study for reviewing familiar concepts and group study for learning new content areas.

What will likely be different now from your earlier study experiences in high school or college is the amount of time you have available for study. Looking back, those earlier days were a lot easier when you had fewer commitments. As you prepare for your certification examination you must balance your other commitments (e.g., family, work) with your need to prepare for the examination.

Plan the best time for taking the examination. If you know that the next few months are especially busy for you with unusual work expectations (e.g., staff shortages, preparing for an accreditation visit) or family responsibilities (e.g., vacation, childcare, holidays), don't add to these burdens by scheduling the examination during that period. Remember, you have the flexibility to choose a testing time that works best for you.

Because the CNOR certification examination is available Monday through Saturday throughout the year, register and schedule the examination at a time that is best for you — a time that allows you adequate preparation and no other major commitments or conflicts. Please visit the CCI website (www.cc-institute.org) for current testing deadlines and windows.

Remember, this certification examination is important for you both personally and professionally. Once you have made the commitment to take the examination, commit also to developing a personalized study plan — and stick to it! Engage help from your family, friends, and colleagues to stick to your study plan.

Question #4 — How do I plan and manage my study time?

Once you have completed your learning needs assessment and identified what you need to study, you will be able to develop a study schedule that, if adhered to, should guide you to a successful testing experience. Study to your weaknesses. Obviously, the more knowledge weaknesses you identify in major areas that will be covered on the CNOR certification examination, the greater time you will need to allow for fulfilling your study schedule.

Most important is to stay focused and committed to your study plan. You will be most confident if you plan for your study time and stick to the study schedule you develop. Use your study time wisely. Make use of any spare time that you have to review concepts.

Here are some suggestions to make the best use of your study time.

- Make a timeline, based on the date for your examination, which outlines specific daily and weekly study time commitments and goals. Make sure your timeline takes into account personal lifestyle issues (work schedule, holidays, family responsibilities, etc.) that will impact the time available to study.

- Set a study schedule and stick with it. Use the study plan found in Appendix A (pages 269-279) to help you organize your time. Engage the help of friends and family to help you stay focused and motivated.

- Prepare a work area where you can leave your study materials so that they are readily available.

- Try to study a little every day, instead of long sessions sporadically; you'll retain more, and it gives you more opportunities to review the material. Repetition is important for learning. Even a few "extra" moments can be useful for your study.

Question #5 — What do I study?

A list of recommended references is found in the study plan and in the introduction to this book. Don't forget online resources that provide additional sources of study materials. There are excellent resources that can be found through the Internet. Consider combining your study preparation with earning continuing education credit. Complete continuing education programs that can be found online, or simply call up a topic of interest and search the Internet to see what is available.

Handy Study Tips

- Consider making flashcards out of index cards and carry those with you everywhere. That way, even an extra five minutes can be turned into valuable study time.

- Balance "old" learning with "new" learning. As you prepare for the examination, you will find some content areas where you need to simply review or "brush up" on your knowledge. In other cases, you may discover "new" content areas that you will need to learn. Remember that the examination is a general examination of perioperative nursing, and the content areas evaluated by the examination may include areas in which you have not previously worked. Try to balance your study sessions to allow some new knowledge gains along with the review of more familiar content.

- Use your work setting as your personal learning lab. In some ways, each workday provides you with an excellent opportunity to prepare for the examination. See how you can build in new knowledge in your daily activities. For example, are you administering a drug that is not used frequently? Use that opportunity to go to a reference and learn more about the drug. Are you assisting in a new surgical procedure? Ask questions of your colleagues and find out all you can, especially about areas that are less familiar to you.

- Let your work colleagues know that you are preparing for your certification examination. Sharing your plans to take the certification examination with your work colleagues will accomplish two purposes. First, ask them to "remind" you that you need to prepare for the examination. Your colleagues can be a great source of support and encouragement. Give them the "okay" to ask you if you are on schedule with your preparation. Second, ask your colleagues to become your study coaches. Remind them to seek you out when they have an interesting surgical case or when there is a new learning opportunity. You may want to share with your colleagues the areas where you believe you have knowledge weaknesses so they can be on the alert for study opportunities that relate.

Stay focused on your goal. At some point in your study cycle, you will no doubt ask yourself, "Why did I decide to do this?" It is normal to feel a bit overwhelmed, but sticking to your goal will be rewarding.

Components of a Multiple-Choice Test Question

In addition to a planned study program, you should work to develop your knowledge and skill in answering multiple-choice questions. It is important that you understand the structure and format of this type of test question.

The CNOR certification examination is comprised of multiple-choice questions. Experts in perioperative nursing write and review the questions of the CNOR certification examination. As such, each question is written to assess important knowledge and skills essential for competent perioperative nursing practice. Much effort goes into developing each question, including multiple reviews by many subject matter experts. Questions are never designed to "trick" the test taker. Rather, questions are designed to be straightfoward and to differentiate test takers who know the content from those who do not.

Each question on the examination is a four-option, multiple-choice test question (or item). A multiple-choice test question consists of the stem and the options. The stem provides the information that supports the question that is being asked. It should contain sufficient information for you to understand what is being asked, even by just reading it alone.

The stem is followed by four options, one of which is the correct answer (or key) as determined by a panel of content experts and validated by current literature. The other three options are the distracters, which are plausible but not correct answers. There is one and only one correct answer among the options provided.

The stem of each test question may be closed-ended or open-ended. A closed-ended question asks a complete question and ends with a question mark. An open-ended question is a type of fill-in-the-blank with the four choices provided as the options. Each of the choices will complete the statement.

The following are examples of each question format:

Closed-ended question:

Which of the following is the rationale for having perioperative nursing personnel immunized with hepatitis B vaccine?
1. Current legislation requires the immunization.
2. Occupational risk of acquiring the hepatitis virus is high. *(Correct answer)*
3. The immunization also provides protection against other forms of hepatitis.
4. Standard precautions require routine immunization for all bloodborne viruses.

Open-ended question:

Perioperative nursing personnel should receive hepatitis B immunization because:
1. current legislation requires the immunization.
2. the occupational risk of acquiring the hepatitis virus is high. *(Correct answer)*
3. the immunization also provides protection against other forms of hepatitis.
4. standard precautions require routine immunization for all bloodborne viruses.

The multiple-choice test questions used in the CNOR certification examination measure either basic knowledge or pose a situation where an application of the knowledge is required. Because clinical practice requires the ability to apply principles and facts to patient situations, most of the test questions on the CNOR certification examination are at the application level. The following are examples of these two types of questions:

Knowledge/Comprehension:

The loss of heat from exposed body parts due to exposure of air currents is known as:
1. evaporation.
2. conduction.

3. radiation.
4. convection. *(Correct answer)*

Application:

During skin preparation, the scrub person informs the perioperative nurse that the sleeve of a student's warm-up jacket has brushed against the area being prepared. Which of the following would be an appropriate response for the perioperative nurse to take first?
1. Report the incident to the instructor for followup.
2. Have the student review the required technique.
3. Review skin preparation at the next in-service program.
4. Inform the student immediately of the break in technique. *(Correct answer)*

Before any question is added to the CNOR certification examination, it is "pretested" on a representative group of test takers to ensure that the question is clearly stated, that there is only one correct answer, and that the question performs statistically across all candidates as intended. Test takers never know which questions are to be scored and which ones are "pretest" questions; therefore, each test taker answers each question presented assuming each question will contribute to the final score on the exam. This process occurs before the question is included and scored in an actual test administration.

One point is given for each correct answer. The total score on the examination is the total points given for all correct answers. There is no penalty for guessing, so be sure to answer all questions. Be cognizant of the time allowed for the test and budget your time wisely so that you can review your answers and complete the entire test within the time allocated.

Taking the CNOR Certification Examination

The CNOR certification examination is a computer-based test that is administered at a test center. Each testing candidate schedules an individualized testing appointment for a date and time that is convenient for him/her. Unlike paper-and-pencil tests where there may be several hundred individuals in the same room, the computer test center is designed to accommodate multiple tests and each person in the testing room may be taking a different examination. Some of these examinations may be shorter or longer than the CNOR certification examination, so you will notice other test takers entering and leaving the room while you are taking your examination.

When the examination begins, you will be presented with a confidentiality statement that acknowledges your agreement to keep the contents of the examination confidential. You may not talk about the test with colleagues nor share any of the test questions. Earning certification should be based on competency, not pre-knowledge of content shared among unscrupulous individuals.

You will next be presented with a brief on-screen tutorial that will orient you to taking a test on a computer. Remember that you do not need computer skills or familiarity with a computer to take the CNOR certification examination. And, even if you are very skilled in using a computer, the tutorial that is part of the examination will teach you how to navigate within this examination.

While the mouse is more commonly used, the keyboard is enabled for use in answering questions. In addition, the tutorial will provide instructions on using the various features: "Previous," which allows you to return to a previously seen question; "Mark," which allows you to identify specific test questions that you would like to return to at a later time whether you have answered the question or skipped it; and "Review," which presents a list of all of the test questions and highlights those questions that you have marked. As you proceed through the test, you may skip a question and return to it later to answer. You may review questions at any time, or wait until the end of the test. Be sure to answer all the questions before you end your examination session.

You should complete the tutorial in its entirety, focusing on how the features of the test operate so that you are familiar with these functions. Your answers to the practice questions in the tutorial are not included in your test score.

The test center staff that proctors the examination and monitors your activities will be located in a viewing area outside the testing room and are available if you need assistance. They are not content experts about perioperative nursing, so they are not able to provide you with any assistance about the test questions themselves. Their role is to monitor the activities in the testing room and report any unusual situations or inappropriate behavior. If you have a concern about a test question, you will have an opportunity to report your concern at the end of the examination by completing an online survey of your testing experience.

You will find more information about the testing situation in the *CNOR Candidate Handbook*. In addition, your Authorization to Test (ATT) that will be sent to you includes instructions about the day of the examination, what time to arrive at the testing center, what identification you will need, and other general guidelines.

Hints for Taking Tests

For many individuals, the CNOR certification examination will be the first test taken in many years. The mere thought of sitting for four hours answering multiple-choice questions brings back memories of earlier testing situations. So it is important that you prepare yourself to be in the best physical and mental condition that is possible.

If you have not taken a computer-based test before, search out opportunities to practice using this method. Many hospitals' annual competencies are computer-based. Many continuing education evaluations are also computer-based. And there are many practice tests available online.

Keep yourself in good physical health before the examination date. You should plan to eat a balanced meal the evening before and then get a good night's sleep. Sleep rather than cram the night before; your critical thinking skills are not based solely on the information you've memorized. Plan to eat breakfast before a morning appointment (or lunch before an afternoon appointment), because you will be in the testing room for over four hours. Avoid over-eating though, as too much food or liquids could make you tired. Feeling well and being rested are important strategies for success. You need to be able to read carefully and think clearly.

Some people become anxious about the testing situation and have difficulty focusing and processing complex information. One way to reduce this anxiety is for you to identify those portions of the exam day that are completely in your control. Be sure you know the directions to the testing center and leave ample time for traffic delays. Know where you will park if you are driving yourself to the test site. Make certain that the required admissions materials are collected the evening before (see "Day of Test Checklist") and are readily available to you as you leave for your appointment.

Test-Taking Guidelines

Success in passing the certification examination takes more than just knowing the content. You need to understand how to read and answer multiple-choice test questions. There is a very simple and easy-to-follow strategy in taking multiple-choice tests.

When reading multiple-choice test questions, it is important to remember that there is one and only one correct answer. So, consider the following.

- Attempt to answer the question before reading the options, and then look for an option that best fits your answer. You should be able to answer a multiple-choice question without reading the options.

- Cover up the options and see if you can determine an answer to the question being asked. Then, uncover the options. Often you will find that your answer is one of the options provided. In that case, your best course of action is to go with your first answer. Try to avoid changing an answer.

- Note that the options are written to be plausible to those who do not know the content. Well-written multiple-choice questions are designed to have four plausible options. The intent is to discriminate between those candidates who know the information and those who do not. If you are unsure of the answer, try to eliminate options that you believe are incorrect. This improves your chance of selecting the correct answer.

- Eliminate options that have absolutes, such as "always" or "never." There is very little in nursing practice that is absolute. Most courses of action in clinical practice and most client responses are "usually" or "generally."

- Read the question carefully, paying special attention to phrases such as "most," "most appropriate," "primarily," "first," and "initially." Often, all of the options are applicable to the situation, but only one option fits the emphasis included in the stem.

- Answer all of the questions. Credit is given for all correct answers. So if you are unsure of an answer, take an educated guess among the plausible options.

- Monitor your progress by noting the time remaining on the computer screen. The CNOR certification examination is timed to provide you with about one minute per question. If you find that you are taking more time than expected to answer a question, mark the question and return to it once you have finished reading through the entire test. You do not want to spend too much time reading one test question and then run out of time, leaving several questions at the end unanswered. Unanswered questions will be scored as incorrect.

- Review your work after you have completed the test. Once you have read through the test and answered as many questions as you can, you should return to review the questions that you may have skipped or marked for further review. Then, if there is available time when you have completed the entire test, you can review all of the questions and reconsider your choices. You should refrain from making too many changes. Often, test takers change a right response to a wrong response.

How to Avoid Making Errors

Being successful in passing the certification examination requires that you also avoid making mistakes in answering the test questions. One helpful strategy to avoid test-taking errors is to take practice tests. Become familiar with the format of multiple-choice questions. Use the CNOR practice tests as a method of improving your knowledge and identifying areas for further study.

When answering practice questions, consider the following as methods to avoid making testing errors:

- Read each question carefully. Errors are made when you do not read the question carefully and completely. Look for and identify the important points involved with the question. Read each option carefully, noting which option most closely matches the intent of the question. Eliminate the options that are not correct and choose the best response that addresses the question being asked.

- Assume that all of the information you need is presented in the test question. The stem of a multiple-choice test question should contain all of the information that is necessary for the test taker to answer the question. When you read the question, avoid the common pitfall of "reading into" the question. Doing this may only confuse you. If certain patient characteristics, such as age, diagnosis, clinical setting, or other related information, are important to know to answer the question, they will be provided.

Otherwise, answer the question from the perspective of the most common situation.

• Identify content areas where your knowledge base is weak. Use the practice test as an opportunity to evaluate your current knowledge of perioperative nursing. When you answer questions incorrectly, use the opportunity to learn the reasons for the incorrect answers. Ask yourself, "Why was my choice wrong?" The best way to learn the content is to understand the underlying rationale for the correct as well as the incorrect answers.

• Understand the basic intent of the test question. One of the most common errors that test takers make is not understanding the intent of the question. Is the question asking for you to make a decision about identifying a priority, a sequence of events, or an important patient presentation? Often in these types of questions, all of the options are plausible for the situation, but the correct answer is the one that is most important, has the highest priority, or is the first action to be taken. Look for the guiding words that give you the direction or emphasis to take.

Day-of-Test Checklist

Within 24 hours before the examination, you should:

• Avoid engaging in any known stressful events. Many of us know what events tend to cause us stress. If at all possible, try to avoid engaging in or attending events that are known stressors just before taking the examination. Practice using relaxation methods to create a calm mental perspective about the test. This will enable you to think clearly and problem solve the questions.

• Obtain sufficient rest and sleep. Fatigue and lethargy will only inhibit your thinking and problem-solving abilities. Engage in any sleep rituals that tend to promote your sleeping ability.

• Limit use of any stimulants, including coffee. Stimulants will affect your ability to receive sufficient rest and sleep. Avoid taking any stimulants, including coffee, late in the day and before bedtime the night before the test.

• Review the CNOR confirmation packet with regard to your responsibilities on the day of the examination. It is your responsibility to be aware of the rules and regulations regarding the CNOR testing experience. If you do not follow the rules as outlined in the confirmation packet, you can be denied access to the testing center. After all of your studying and planning, you do not want to forfeit your testing opportunity at the last minute.

• Arrive at the testing center at least 30 minutes before your test appointment. If you are unsure of the exact location of the test center, it is strongly suggested that you locate the test center ahead of time. Determine how long it will take you to drive there or go by public transportation, if applicable, by following the route before the day of your test. The test center can provide you with directions if you need them or go on-line and print out directions. Unforeseen and uncontrollable events, such as accidents or inclement weather, can cause delays in your travel time. It is far better to arrive early than to be late and miss your appointment.

• Limit the personal items you bring with you. You will not be permitted to take hand-bags, wallets, books, watches. cellular phones, laptops, or any other personal belong-ings into the testing room. The test center has lockers where you can store any items you bring. The proctor will provide you with scrap paper. There is no space at the test center for family members or friends to accompany you to your testing appoint-ment. There will be a check-in process at the test center before you go into the testing room. Pockets must be emptied and no materials are allowed in the testing room.

• Make sure that you bring the following items with you to the test center:

☐ Authorization to Test: This letter informs the test center staff of your eligbility to test, your name, and the test that you are taking.

☐ One form of current, government-issued photo identification, such as a driver's license or a passport, with a signature. Be sure your identification matches exactly the name on your Authorization to Test.

After the Examination

Try to avoid "second guessing." While it is common practice to "relive" the test experi-ence, try not to second guess the responses you gave to each test question. Without the content of the question directly in front of you, it is too easy to "conclude" you may have answered incorrectly.

Do not share information about the test or test questions. Remember that you have signed a pledge to keep the contents of the CNOR certification examination confidential. Sharing information about the test or discussing specific questions about the test with colleagues or other test takers violates this confidentiality pledge. In addition, multiple forms of the examination are being administered so it is highly likely that the questions you saw on your test will not be the exact same questions another test taker saw.

Summary

Success occurs when you have made a detailed plan for preparing for the examination and have stuck to it! Essential components of success include:
• Identifying knowledge areas for review.
• Understanding the testing process.
• Being confident that your study habits have prepared you to be successful.

Self-Assessment for the CNOR Exam

CCI wants to help prepare you for success in seeking the professional credential for perioperative registered nurses (CNOR). The following self-assessment tool may be used to determine readiness for taking the exam, identify areas of strength and needed improvement, and aid in the development of a test preparation plan.

1. Have I met the criteria for eligibility to take the exam?

   Yes   No

   □   □   Currently licensed as an RN in the country where currently practicing perioperative nursing.

   □   □   Have a minimum of 2 years and 2,400 hours of perioperative practice in an administrative, teaching, research, or general staff capacity.

   □   □   Currently working either part- or full-time in a perioperative role.

   > *Please check the CCI website (www.cc-institute.org) for the most current eligibility requirements. CCI reserves the right to change eligibility requirements at any time.*

2. Does my day-to-day practice involve a variety of surgical procedures, specialties, and patient age groups, or is my role restricted to one or two specialties or age groups?

   My current practice involves the following types of cases:

   _____

   _____

   _____

   _____

   I will need additional exposure/information on the following types of cases:

   _____

   _____

   _____

   _____

3. Do I perform my own preoperative assessment, or do I mostly rely on documentation from admitting personnel in developing my plan of care?

4. Do I know the action, dose, side effects, and contraindications for the medications my patient is taking pre-procedure?

   □ Yes   □ No

5. Do I know the action, dose, route, side effects, and contraindications for the medications that are administered during the intraoperative period?

   □ Yes   □ No

6. Do I have access to Central Processing personnel and resources?

   □ Yes   □ No

7. Do I participate in hand-offs to PACU nurses, or does someone else give report to the RN?

8. Is my facility current on Joint Commission, CMS, and other regulatory standards?

   □ Yes   □ No

9. Are Association of periOperative Registered Nurses (AORN) standards and recommended practices cited in my facility's policies and procedures?
    □ Yes   □ No

10. Do I incorporate the most current AORN standards and recommended practices into my practice?
    □ Yes   □ No

11. Are my facility's policies and procedures updated to reflect current best practice?
    □ Yes   □ No

12. Does my facility library/unit manager/educator have access to current reference and resource materials (e.g., *Perioperative Standards and Recommended Practices, Alexander's Care of the Patient in Surgery, Berry and Kohn's Operating Room Technique)*?
    □ Yes   □ No

13. Have I provided myself with adequate time to study (typically 3 months) prior to taking the exam?
    □ Yes   □ No

14. Have I reviewed the *CCI Candidate Handbook* (found at www.cc-institute.org) to familiarize myself with the testing process?
    □ Yes   □ No

15. Do I have a mentor or resource person who understands the certification process?
    □ Yes Person's name: _____   □ No
            Contact info: _____

16. Does my facility have a CCI Champion? (go to www.cc-institute.org for a list of Champions)
    □ Yes   Champion's name: _____   □ No

17. I have identified and put a plan in place to address barriers to preparation for the exam:
    □ Cost of exam
    □ Cost of study materials
    □ Facility support/reward/recognition
    □ Time
    □ Testing anxiety

Step Back

Critically analyze the results of your self-assessment. Numerous "no" answers, limited exposure to all components of perioperative nursing (pre-, intra-, and postoperative), and/or specialization to specific types of patients or procedures does not mean you cannot be successful on the exam, but it does suggest participating in additional learning opportunities to address identified deficits.

Learning Needs Assessment

The CNOR exam is based on the following domains, or major topics. The following tool can be used to evaluate your knowledge of items found on the CNOR examination. Together with the self-assessment, this tool provides a baseline for determining preparation needs. For each domain, score your current knowledge based on the following key:

1 — Very Certain: I know this content area well and believe that my work experiences have fully prepared me. I am comfortable with current practices and believe I am up-to-date with new developments and advances.

2 — Certain: I am reasonably comfortable with this content area and believe that my work experiences have prepared me fairly well.

3 — Undecided: I have some knowledge and some experience in this area, but there may be a few content areas where I am not as strong or for which my work experiences have not fully prepared me.

4 — Uncertain: I am aware that I have some knowledge deficits and/or a lack of work experience in this content area. I will need to engage in some study or other remediation to be comfortable with this content area.

5 — Very Uncertain: I am aware that I have many knowledge deficits and/or lack work experiences in this content area. This is an area of weakness for me and one that will require me to remediate before taking the examination.

To help determine what content you will need to review the most, match the percentage of questions in the domain and the areas scored 3, 4, or 5 to help determine what content will need the most review.

Domain	My level of competency	Percentage of questions on the exam
1. Preoperative Patient Assessment and Diagnosis		14%
2. Identify Expected Outcomes and Develop an Individualized Plan of Care		9%
3. Intraoperative Activities		31%
4. Communication		9%
5. Transfer of Care		5%
6. Cleaning, Disinfecting, Packaging, Sterilizing, Transporting, and Storing Instruments and Supplies		12%
7. Emergency Situations		8%
8. Management of Personnel, Services, and Materials		6%
9. Professional Accountability		6%

NOTES

CHAPTER I:
Preoperative Patient Assessment and Diagnosis

> **Test Specifications:**
> *14% of CNOR test questions are based on Preoperative Patient Assessment and Diagnosis.*

Introduction

Patient assessment is the cornerstone of all nursing practice. It is the first item listed in the nursing process, and although perioperative nurses may conduct a more focused assessment than a med-surg or critical care nurse, the more information we gather, the better able we will be to identify special needs (diagnosis), determine our next steps (plan of care), and anticipate what we would like to happen (expected outcomes). The next two chapters provide opportunities to apply what we know to common perioperative situations. A patient-centered approach is utilized for several reasons:

1. The Institute of Medicine has identified this as one of six needed health care competencies (IOM, 2001).

2. Utilizing a patient-centered approach helps keep the focus on patient care, rather than on what an individual nurse would do based on a facility's policies and procedures.

Checklists and preference cards are useful in helping us organize and complete the tasks in the OR in a safe and collaborative manner. However, in developing a plan of care from the *patient's* perspective, it may be more useful to create a concept or mind map (see sample on following page), which is an organizational tool that allows us to look at the connection between our patients' needs and how we meet those needs. It also is a good reminder that events do not necessarily occur in order, and certainly not in isolation; multiple things can and do happen at the same time, and one event can have an impact on many other systems. The concept map will encourage us to view the big picture, ask questions about our patients, and allow us to appreciate the interrelatedness of data obtained from our patient assessment and our plan of care.

There is no one "correct" way to develop a concept map; the samples in the Study Guide Toolbox at http://www.cc-institute/toolbox are examples only and are to be used to help get you started. Feel free to develop your own map. It is more important to develop a tool that you can use and that makes sense to you than to strictly follow the examples. Although they may be arranged differently, you will find that the main components of your map will be the same as those found in the learning activities.

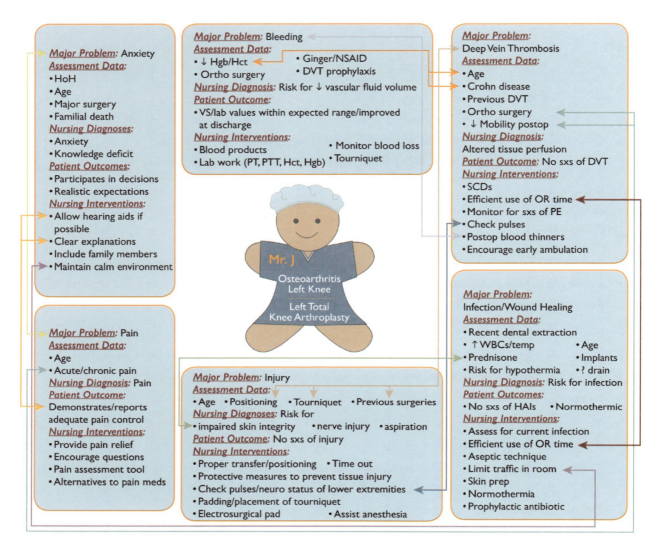

Case Study

To encourage continuity in learning activities between pre-, intra-, and postoperative patient care, a case study approach will be presented in Chapters 1, 2, 3, 5, and 8. Our imaginary patient will guide us through critical thinking exercises that can be applied to any patient, of any age, and for any procedure. Templates for forms are included in the Toolbox at http://www.cc-institute/toolbox for you to make multiple copies as you wish in developing your own plans of care.

The case study for this *Guide* is presented on the following two pages. Case study activities presented in this and later chapters appear in a box with an orange border as shown on the next page.

Case Study

Note: *This case study will be used for activities in Chapters 1, 2, 3, 5, and 8.*

Your first patient of the day is Mr. J., who is scheduled for a left total knee arthroplasty at 0730. You assist the scrub person in opening the room and then go to AM Admissions to meet your patient. After reviewing Mr. J.'s medical record and conducting your preoperative interview, you have obtained the following information:

Chief Complaint:
Osteoarthritis, left knee.
Knee grates, "catches," and is painful after exercise.
X-ray left knee shows bone-on-bone.

Past Medical History:
Thyroid cancer, diagnosed 1996
Hiatal hernia, diagnosed 1998
Crohn disease, diagnosed 2011
DVT following total hip arthroplasty, resolved with warfarin without further complications

Past Surgical History:
Near total thyroidectomy, 1996
Laparoscopic Nissen fundoplication, 1998
Bilateral cataract removal with intraocular lens implant, 1998
Small bowel resection, 2011
Left total hip arthroplasty, 2012
Full mouth dental extraction 5 days ago because of decaying teeth

Family History:
Parents deceased
Maternal grandfather died during surgery secondary to thyroid complications.

Social:
Patient is retired schoolteacher. He is widowed. He has three grown children, the closest of whom lives 200 miles away. He considers himself fairly active. He quit smoking 15 years ago. He rarely drinks alcohol. He has a signed Medical Durable Power of Attorney with his daughter listed as his agent.

Allergies:
NKDA
Allergic to shellfish (nausea, vomiting, rash)

Continued on following page.

Case Study, *continued*

Medications:
Levothyroxine — 250 mcg/day, last dose yesterday AM
Ibuprofen — 400 mg PRN for knee pain, last dose last night
Ginger — 1 capsule every morning for "indigestion"
Prednisone — 25 mg/day for Crohn's flare-up; last dose yesterday AM

Physical Exam:
85-year-old male in no acute distress
DP and PT peripheral pulses 3+ bilaterally
Wears hearing aids bilaterally
Full set of dentures in place
Ht — 5'9"   Wt — 179 pounds
Vital signs

BP — 138/80 mmHg	T (TM) — 100° F
P — 48 bpm	R — 16/min
Pulse ox — 95% on room air	Pain — 3/10

Diagnostic Tests and Lab Values:

Hematology	Reference range*
WBCs — 11,300/mm³	5,000-10,000/mm³
RBCs — 5.07 x 10¹²/mm³	4.7-6.14 x 10¹²/mm³
Hemoglobin — 14.4 g/dL	14.0-18.0 g/dL
Hematocrit — 42.7%	42-52%
Na+ — 143 mEq/L	136-145 mEq/L
K+ — 4.8 mEq/L	3.5-5.0 mEq/L
TSH — 0.01 mU/L	2-10 mU/L
CO₂ — 29 mEq/L	23-30 mEq/L
Cl- — 107 mEq/L	98-106 mEq/L
Blood glucose — Fasting 90 mg/dL	70-110 mg/dL
Ca++ — 8.4 mg/dL	9.0-10.5 mg/dL
BUN — 20 mg/dL	10-20 mg/dL
Creatinine, blood — 1.2 mg/dL	0.6-1.2 mg/dL
Protein serum — 5.8 g/dL	6.4-8.3 g/dL
Platelets — 259,000/mm³	150,000-400,000/mm³

Chest x-ray: Normal age-related changes; chest clear to auscultation.
IV: D5 ½ NS infusing at 100 mL/hr in dorsum right hand; no swelling or redness noted.
Sequential compression stocking on right leg.

*Reference: Pagana, K.D., & Pagana, T.J. (2013). *Mosby's Manual of Diagnostic & Laboratory Tests* (11th ed.). St. Louis: Mosby Elsevier.

Module 1: Assess the Health Status of the Patient

Patient assessment involves the continuous collection of subjective and objective data from a variety of sources. This information is then used to develop nursing diagnoses, which will drive the plan of care.

Competency Outcomes

To successfully complete the activities in this module, you will need to be able to:

1. Differentiate normal from abnormal anatomy and physiology based on age-related factors.
2. Integrate components of relevant pathophysiologic processes (concurrent disease processes, inflammatory/immune responses, etc.) into a surgical patient plan of care.
3. Collect, analyze, and prioritize patient data (allergies, lab values, EKG, arterial blood gas results, other medical conditions, previous relevant surgical history, NPO status) from a variety of sources (chart review, patient/family interview, consultation with other health care team members).
4. Conduct an individualized physical assessment.
5. Select nursing diagnoses based on data collected during the preoperative assessment period.
6. Demonstrate cultural competence in assessing needs for a diverse patient population.
7. Provide for continuity in patient care through effective interdisciplinary communication.

Recommended Readings

Alexander's Care of the Patient in Surgery. (2015, 15th ed.), Chapter 1: Concepts basic to perioperative nursing; Unit II: Surgical interventions.

Berry and Kohn's Operating Room Technique. (2013, 12th ed.), Chapter 2: Foundations of perioperative patient care standards; Chapter 7: The patient: The reason for your existence; Chapter 8: Perioperative pediatrics; Chapter 9: Perioperative geriatrics; Chapter 11: Ambulatory surgery centers and alternative surgical locations; Chapter 21: Preoperative preparation of the patient; Chapter 25: Coordinated roles of the scrub person and the circulating nurse.

Perioperative Standards and Recommended Practices. (2014), Section 1: Standards of perioperative nursing practice; Recommended practices for minimally invasive surgery.

Key Words

Age specific, assessment, diagnostic studies, laboratory results, nursing diagnosis, nursing process, patient education, *Perioperative Nursing Data Set* (PNDS), physical assessment, preoperative testing

Patient Assessment

Importance of Assessment

The first step in the nursing process, assessment, is performed throughout the patient's entire health care experience. The initial assessment identifies baseline values and actual or potential problems through information provided by the patient, family and guardians, significant others, the medical record, lab work, and other health care providers. This information will be used to formulate perioperative nursing diagnoses and the patient's plan of care, reinforcing the need to both obtain and accurately interpret data.

Components of the Patient Assessment

Rather than a head-to-toe or complete review of systems, perioperative nurses typically perform a more focused patient assessment based on data found in the history and physical and patient interview that are directly applicable to the proposed operative or invasive procedure.

Documentation of Assessment Findings

Whether electronic or paper, to ensure continuity of care the results of the assessment must be documented. Many facilities have preprinted forms, which serve as excellent reminders of components that need to be included in the assessment and help to decrease errors or omissions in the assessment process. Although checklists and boxes are convenient and efficient, all records should have the capability of allowing the nurse to add additional information to reflect a patient's unique needs, as this information is especially important in developing an individualized plan of care. Patients may reveal important information to the nurse that they did not relay to other health care providers; this could affect the surgical procedure or the type of anesthesia planned. Documentation of the patient's assessment should include findings of the focused exam and patient interview.

Activity — Fill in the Blank

1. What sources of data will you use during Mr. J.'s assessment?

_____

_____

_____

_____

_____

_____

_____

2. Which systems will be most important to assess during Mr. J.'s preoperative interview?

_____

_____

_____

_____

_____

_____

"Go To" Case Study Activity
Draw Your Own Concept Map

Go to the Concept Map file in the Study Guide Toolbox at http://www.cc-institute. org/toolbox. Using the patient information on pages 35-36, follow the instructions to begin drawing your concept map. The steps involved in organizing the data are repeated here for your convenience.

Put your patient's name, preoperative diagnosis, and proposed procedure in the center of the map.

Make a list of all the data you feel you will need to address in your plan of care.

Identify Mr. J.'s "major problems." Some of these are typical for every surgery (e.g., infection, pain, anxiety), while others will be specific for Mr. J. Eventually these will turn into nursing diagnoses; for now, just label them with whatever terms you're comfortable using. Put each "major problem" into its own box.

Arrange the assessment data from your list under their corresponding "major problems" boxes. The same data may be used in multiple boxes.

What critical information needs to be communicated to the following health care team members?

Anesthesia provider:

Surgeon:

Scrub person:

Case Study Activity — Critical Thinking

The following are common risk factors for infection. Based on your preoperative assessment of Mr. J., circle the items that put him at risk for a postoperative infection.

Poorly controlled diabetes   Nutritional status   Gingivitis/dental health

Obesity   Age   Existing infection   Altered immune system   Smoking

Activity — Matching

Match the patient assessment items on the left with the corresponding nursing intervention on the right. Note: Some items will have multiple answers. Answers may be used more than once.

Assessment Data:

Identification of patient _____

Baseline vital signs (temperature, pulse, respirations, blood pressure, pulse oximetry reading, and pain assessment) _____

Height and weight _____

Known medical conditions _____

Prescription and over-the-counter medications, supplements including herbal preparations taken on a routine basis, and last medication administration _____

Allergies or sensitivities, including latex and food _____

NPO status _____

Previous surgical history, including asking about metal implants and untoward reactions to anesthesia _____

Skin condition _____

Level of consciousness _____

Emotional status _____

Risk for falling _____

Any history of drug or alcohol abuse _____

Smoking history (packs per day and pack years) _____

Signs of physical or emotional abuse _____

Diagnostic test results _____

Diversity and cultural needs _____

Knowledge deficits related to surgery/recovery _____

Intervention:

A. Positioning

B. Patient education/communication

C. Medication and solution administration

D. Moving/transfer

E. Infection prevention

F. Adequate airway/oxygen exchange

G. Maintenance of skin integrity

H. Preventing wrong site, wrong patient, wrong procedure

I. Normothermia

J. Adequate tissue perfusion

Activity — Critical Thinking

Read the following sentence, and then count the number of "f's" in the sentence.

Finished files are the result of years of scientific study combined with the experience of years.

How many did you count?

"Go To" Activity — Check It Out!

In the Study Guide Toolbox at http://www.cc-institute.org/toolbox, go to Question #6, NPO Status, and Question #10, Hyperglycemia, under the Perioperative question of the week tab for additional critical-thinking questions.

"Go To" Activity — Skill Building

Compare your facility's policy and procedure on length of time for preoperative fasting with the American Society of Anesthesiologists' recommended guidelines. How do they differ?

Additional Readings/Resources

Bashaw, M., & Scott, D.N. (2012). Surgical risk factors in geriatric perioperative patients. *AORN Journal, 96*(1), 58-74.

Jest, A.D., & Tonge, A. (2011). Using a learning needs assessment to identify knowledge deficits regarding procedural sedation for pediatric patients. *AORN Journal, 94*(6), 567-577.

Munro, C.A. (2010). The development of a pressure ulcer risk-assessment scale for perioperative patients. *AORN Journal, 92*(3), 272-287.

Peterson, C. (2010). Requirement for a history and physical examination before minor surgery. *AORN Journal*, *92*(5), 586-587.

Rutan, L., & Sommers, K. (2012). Hyperglycemia as a risk factor in the perioperative patient. *AORN Journal, 95*(1), 352-364.

Simons, D., & Chabris, C. (2010). Selective attention test: The invisible gorilla. Retrieved Feb. 23, 2014, from www.theinvisiblegorilla.com/videos.html
Note: Make sure to watch both the first and second videos.

Taylor, E. (2009). Providing developmentally based care for school-aged and adolescent patients. *AORN Journal, 90*(2), 261-267.

Module 2: Review of Preoperative Medications

Obtaining a detailed history of current medications and allergies is an excellent way to further understand a patient's overall state of health. Evaluating current medication information, including prescription, over the counter, and herbal/alternative drugs, serves multiple purposes. It identifies allergies; concurrent disease processes and the severity of the condition; the effectiveness of the drug in treating the condition; the patient's knowledge of pharmacology related to his/her medications; and the history of compliance with a drug regimen (which may serve as a predictor for successfully following postoperative instructions). In addition, potential adverse effects and drug interactions between home, perioperative, and discharge medications can be identified early and thereby avoided.

Competency Outcomes

To successfully complete the activities in this module, you will need to be able to:

1. Reconcile current medications (preoperative medications, current prescription drugs, over-the-counter medications, alternative and herbal supplements, and medical marijuana) and alcohol and recreational drug consumption with patient's condition and proposed surgical procedure.
2. Identify possible adverse effects of patient's daily medications on the surgical procedure.

Recommended Readings

Alexander's Care of the Patient in Surgery. (2015, 15th ed.), Chapter 2: Patient safety and risk management; Chapter 30: Integrative health practices: Complementary and alternative therapies.

Berry and Kohn's Operating Room Technique. (2013, 12th ed.), Chapter 2: Foundations of perioperative patient care standards; Chapter 11: Ambulatory surgery centers and alternative surgical locations; Chapter 21: Preoperative preparation of the patient; Chapter 23: Surgical pharmacology, pp. 420-421.

Perioperative Standards and Recommended Practices. (2014), Recommended practices: Medication safety.

Key Words

Allergies, complementary/alternative medicine (CAM), herbs, medication reconciliation, patient/family education, pharmacology, side effects

Case Study Activity — Matching

Match Mr. J.'s current medications to the action from the list on the right:

Levothyroxine _____

Ibuprofen _____

Ginger _____

Prednisone _____

A. steroidal anti-inflammatory

B. nonsteroidal anti-inflammatory

C. complementary treatment for nausea, arthritis

D. suppresses TSH

Case Study Activity — Critical Thinking

How will the use of a tourniquet during Mr. J.'s surgery affect the timing of the dose of his preoperative antibiotic?

Which of Mr. J.'s home medications could influence the surgical procedure? Why?

Additional Readings/Resources

American Society of Anesthesiologists (n.d.). Herbal supplements and anesthesia. Retrieved Feb. 23, 2014, from http://www.lifelinetomodernmedicine.com/Anesthesia-Topics/Herbal-Supplements-and-Anesthesia.aspx. Bonus: Includes a video.

Chard, R. (2009). Medication reconciliation across the continuum of care. *AORN Journal, 92*(4), 470-471.

Eisenstein, D.H. (2012). Anticoagulation management in the ambulatory surgical setting. *AORN Journal, 95*(4), 510-524.

U.S. Department of Health and Human Services, National Institutes of Health. (n.d.). National Center for Complementary and Alternative Medicine (NCCAM). Retrieved Feb. 23, 2014, from http://nccam.nih.gov/

Module 3: Initiation of the Universal Protocol

The Universal Protocol was initiated by The Joint Commission to prevent wrong site, wrong procedure, and wrong person surgery. A standardized checklist that is consistently initiated and followed has been found to help decrease surgical errors.

Competency Outcomes

To successfully complete the activities in this module, you will need to be able to:

1. Implement components of the Universal Protocol.
2. Identify AORN standards and recommended practices that help to prevent adverse outcomes.

Recommended Readings

Alexander's Care of the Patient in Surgery. (2015, 15th ed.), Chapter 2: Patient safety and risk management; Chapter 20: Orthopedic surgery, p. 688.

Berry and Kohn's Operating Room Technique. (2013, 12th ed.), Chapter 2: Foundations of perioperative patient care standards; Chapter 3: Legal, regulatory, and ethical issues.

Key Words

The Joint Commission (TJC), preoperative verification, site marking, wrong person, wrong procedure, wrong site

Activity — Fill in the Blank

What three "wrongs" will implementation of the Universal Protocol help prevent?

1. _____
2. _____
3. _____

Activity — Critical Thinking

Identify the corresponding AORN standard or recommended practice that addresses each of the following "never events."

Answer:

1. Surgery performed on the wrong body part, the wrong patient, or the wrong procedure.   _____

2. Unintended retention of a foreign object in a patient after surgery or other procedure.   _____

3. Patient death or serious disability associated with a medication error.   _____

4. Patient death or serious disability associated with a burn incurred from any source.   _____

5. Hospital acquired pressure ulcers.   _____

6. Deep vein thrombosis.   _____

7. Hospital acquired surgical site infections.   _____

Activity — Mark the Site

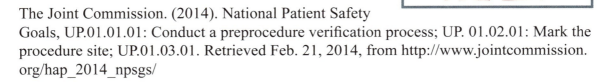

Mark the illustration to correspond with the correct site and side for Mr. J.'s surgery.

Additional Readings/Resources

Conrardy, J.A., Brenek, B., & Myers, S. (2010). Determining the state of knowledge for implementing the Universal Protocol recommendations: An integrative review of the literature. *AORN Journal, 92*(2), 194-207.

Guglielmi, C. (2010). Table talk: Strategies for preventing wrong site, wrong procedure, and wrong patient surgery. *AORN Journal, 92*(1), 22-27.

The Joint Commission. (2014). National Patient Safety Goals, UP.01.01.01: Conduct a preprocedure verification process; UP. 01.02.01: Mark the procedure site; UP.01.03.01. Retrieved Feb. 21, 2014, from http://www.jointcommission.org/hap_2014_npsgs/

Knudson, L. (2013). Time out remains key weapon in fight against wrong-site surgeries. *AORN Journal, 97*(6), C5-C6.

McNamara, S.A. (2012). National Time Out Day: More than "a pause and a checklist." *AORN Journal, 95*(6), 805-814.

Norton, E. (2011). Using an alternative site marking form to comply with the Universal Protocol. *AORN Journal, 93*(5), 600-606.

Norton, E.K., & Rangel, S.J. (2010). Implementing a pediatric surgical safety checklist in the OR and beyond. *AORN Journal, 92*(1), 61-71.

Watson, D.S. (2009). Implementing the Universal Protocol. *AORN Journal, 90*(2), 283-287.

Module 4: Obtaining Surgical Consent

Informed consent is the process of ensuring that a patient understands the benefits, risks, and alternatives to the surgical procedure. It serves as a contract between the patient and the health care practitioner performing the operation or invasive procedure. The signed consent form is one of the primary documents on which the perioperative nurse relies when developing a plan of care.

Competency Outcomes

To successfully complete the activities in this module, you will need to be able to:

1. Identify components of a surgical consent.
2. Define "informed consent."
3. Outline steps for obtaining consent.

Recommended Readings

Alexander's Care of the Patient in Surgery. (2015, 15th ed.), Chapter 2: Patient safety and risk management.

Berry and Kohn's Operating Room Technique. (2013, 12th ed.), Chapter 3: Legal, regulatory, and ethical issues.

Perioperative Standards and Recommended Practices. (2014), Recommended practices; Information Management, pp. 448-449.

> **"Go To" Activity — Check It Out!**
>
> In the Toolbox at http://www.cc-institute/toolbox, go to Question #28, Informed consent and minors, under the Perioperative question of the week tab for an additional critical-thinking question.

Key Words

Alternatives, autonomy, benefits, complications, informed consent, patient rights, privacy, respect, risk

Activity — Fill in the Blank

The surgeon or practitioner performing the procedure is responsible for informing the patient about the proposed procedure in terms that he or she can understand.

It is the _____'s responsibility to obtain informed consent.

Activity — Critical Thinking

How does obtaining surgical consent for a child differ from that of an adult?

Case Study Activity — Consent

Mr. J.'s consent and the surgery schedule read right total knee arthroplasty. Mr. J., the H&P, and knee films all state that the left knee is the correct operative site. How will you address this discrepancy?

"Go To" Activity — Skill Building

Obtain a consent form from your facility. Compare it with the documentation typically included on an informed consent:

- Name of patient
- Name of facility where procedure will be performed
- Surgical procedure
- Site/side as applicable
- Benefits, risks, alternatives
- Person(s) performing the procedure
- Statement that procedure was explained to the patient/legal guardian
- Signature of the patient or legal guardian
- Signature of the surgeon
- Signature of witness
- Date and time consent is obtained
- Additional permissions requested (for example, blood transfusions, presence of visitors/students, photographs)

Additional Readings/Resources

Burlingame, B. (2009). Length of time a signed informed consent is valid. *AORN Journal*, *90*(3), 446-447.

Peterson, C. (2010). Responsibility for obtaining the surgical informed consent. In Clinical issues, *AORN Journal, 92*(5), 585-586.

Woods, K.D. (2012). Clinical issues: Informed consent for repeated procedures; Obtaining informed consent after administration of preoperative sedation. *AORN Journal, 96*(6), 659-662.

Module 5: Ensuring Patients' Rights By Providing Information on Advance Directives, Do-Not-Resuscitate

Patients undergoing an operative or invasive procedure have the same rights in determining the course of their care as any other patient. Clear communication between the patient and the surgical team is even more important, as the nature of the care provided during a procedure may mimic a resuscitative event.

Competency Outcomes

To successfully complete the activities in this module, you will need to be able to:

1. Define the terms "advance directive," "medical power of attorney," and "do-not-resuscitate (DNR)."

2. Describe ramifications of a DNR for a surgical patient.
3. Describe methods for confirming advance directive status or DNR status.

Recommended Readings

Alexander's Care of the Patient in Surgery. (2015, 15th ed.), Chapter 2: Patient safety and risk management.

Berry and Kohn's Operating Room Technique. (2013, 12th ed.), Chapter 3: Legal, regulatory, and ethical issues.

Perioperative Standards and Recommended Practices. (2014), Position statement: Perioperative care of patients with do-not-resuscitate orders; Perioperative explications, 1.4: The right to self-determination.

> ## "Go To" Activity — Check It Out!
>
> Go to Question #8, Patient rights and DNR, under the Perioperative question of the week tab in the Toolbox at http://www.cc-institute/toolbox, for an additional critical-thinking question.

Key Words

Advance directive, allow natural death (AND), CPR directive, do-not-resuscitate (DNR), living will, medical durable power of attorney, Patient Self-Determination Act (PSDA)

Activity — True or False?

Under the Patient Self-Determination Act, patients have the legal right to accept or refuse medical treatment, including resuscitation, even if refusal will likely result in death.

TRUE ____   FALSE ____

> ### "Go To" Activity — Skill Building
>
> What is your facility's policy on DNR for surgical patients? Do you have a separate form that must be filled out? If so, how many of the following choices does it include?
> * suspension of DNR orders.
> * continuation of DNR orders.
> * limited resuscitation with procedure-directed orders.
> * limited resuscitation with goal-directed orders.

> ## Case Study Activity — PSDA
>
> Mr. J. has brought his completed medical durable power of attorney form with him. It states that he does not wish life-sustaining measures for an irreversible condition. He says, "I guess I won't be needing this during my surgery." What is your response?

Additional Readings/Resources

Ball, K. (2009). Do-not-resuscitate orders in surgery: Decreasing the confusion. *AORN Journal, 89*(1), 140-150.

Girard, N.J. (2010). Wrongful resuscitation. *AORN Journal, 92*(6), 710, 631.

Physician Orders for Life-Sustaining Treatment Paradigm (POLST). (2012). Retrieved Jan. 21, 2014, from http://www.polst.org/
Note: Provides information on end-of-life planning.

U.S. Department of Health and Human Services. (2008, Aug.). Advance directives and advance care planning: Report to Congress. Retrieved Jan. 21, 2014, from http://aspe.hhs.gov/daltcp/reports/2008/ADCongRpt.pdf

Zinn, J.L. (2012). Do-Not-Resuscitate orders: Providing safe care while honoring the patient's wishes. *AORN Journal, 96*(1), 90-94.

Module 6: Pain Assessment

The importance of pain assessment is reflected by the fact that it is now being considered the "fifth vital sign." An initial baseline pain assessment obtained preoperatively is necessary as signs and symptoms of both acute and chronic pain may be masked by the medications given during the intraoperative period.

Competency Outcomes

To successfully complete the activities in this module, you will need to be able to:

1. Assess a patient for signs and symptoms of pain, taking into account variations related to age, gender, and culture.
2. Utilize a pain-rating scale in assessing a patient's level of pain.
3. Incorporate pain-relief interventions into a plan of care.

Recommended Readings

Alexander's Care of the Patient in Surgery. (2015, 15th ed.), Chapter 5: Anesthesia; Chapter 10: Postoperative patient care and pain management; Chapter 26: Pediatric surgery; Chapter 27: Geriatric surgery; Chapter 30: Integrative health practices: Complementary and alternative therapies.

Berry and Kohn's Operating Room Technique. (2013, 12th ed.), Chapter 8: Perioperative pediatrics; Chapter 30: Postoperative patient care.

Key Words

Analgesia, narcotics, nonsteroidal anti-inflammatories (NSAIDS), nonpharmacologic interventions, opioids, pain assessment, pain block, pain intensity scales, patient-controlled analgesia (PCA), pharmacology, regional anesthesia, self-report, signs, symptoms, The Joint Commission (TJC)

Activity — Matching

Match the most appropriate pain rating scale to the patient described below. (Answers may be used more than once.)

3-year-old girl_____   A. 0-10 Numeric pain intensity scale

45-year-old man _____   B. FACES Pain rating scale

23-year-old woman who   C. Simple descriptive pain intensity scale
does not speak English _____

Case Study Activity — Pain Assessment

While discussing Mr. J.'s pain management plan, he tells you, "I don't plan on taking any of that stuff; I don't want to get addicted." What is your response?

Additional Readings/Resources

Hicks, R.W., Hernandez, J., & Wanzer, L.J. (2012). Perioperative pharmacology: Patient-controlled analgesia. *AORN Journal, 95*(2), 255-265.

Trudeau, J.D., Lamb, E., Gowans, M., & Lauder, G. (2009). A prospective audit of post-operative pain control in pediatric patients. *AORN Journal, 90*(4), 531-542.
Note: This article provides a nice description of another pain rating tool, FLACC (Face, Legs, Activity, Cry, Consolability).

Veteran's Health Administration. (2009). VHA Directive 2009-053: Pain management. Retrieved Feb. 23, 2014, from http://www.va.gov/PAINMANAGEMENT/docs/VHA09PainDirective.pdf

Wright, I. (2011). Peripheral nerve blocks in the outpatient surgery setting. *AORN Journal, 94*(1), 59-77.

Module 7: Development of Nursing Diagnoses

A nursing diagnosis sorts assessment data into real or potential patient problems. Standardized terminology is used to "label" the problem, which enhances clear communication and documentation among members of the health care team. Nursing interventions specific to each diagnosis are then identified. Experience level determines the speed with which a practitioner moves through these steps.

Competency Outcomes

To successfully complete the activities in this module, you will need to be able to:

1. Identify common perioperative nursing diagnoses.
2. Formulate nursing diagnoses that are consistent with the patient's assessment data.

Recommended Readings

Alexander's Care of the Patient in Surgery. (2015, 15th ed.), Chapter 1: Concepts basic to perioperative nursing.

Berry and Kohn's Operating Room Technique. (2013, 12th ed.), Chapter 2: Foundations of perioperative patient care standards.

Key Words

Diagnosis, medical diagnosis, nursing diagnosis, nursing process, *Perioperative Nursing Data Set* (PNDS)

Frequently Used Nursing Diagnoses

Acute pain
Anxiety
Chronic pain
Deficient knowledge
Fear
Hyperthermia
Hypothermia
Imbalanced nutrition
Impaired gas exchange
Impaired transfer ability
Ineffective breathing pattern
Ineffective health maintenance

Nausea
Risk for aspiration
Risk for deficient fluid volume
Risk for electrolyte imbalance
Risk for imbalanced body temperature
Risk for imbalanced fluid volume
Risk for impaired skin integrity
Risk for infection
Risk for injury
Risk for latex allergy response
Risk for perioperative positioning injury
Risk for peripheral neurovascular dysfunction

Source: AORN. (2011). *Perioperative Nursing Data Set* (3rd ed., p. 416). Denver: AORN, Inc.

"Go To" Case Study Activity — Nursing Diagnoses

From your interpretation of Mr. J.'s assessment data, formulate nursing diagnoses to address each identified problem or potential problem. Write your nursing diagnoses in the boxes next to your "major problem" in your concept map in the Study Guide Toolbox at http://www.cc-institute.org/toolbox. Not all of your "major problems" may have a corresponding nursing diagnosis.

Activity — Matching

Match the term with its definition.

Etiology _____

Nursing diagnosis _____

Nursing intervention _____

Problem _____

Sign _____

Symptom _____

A. Objective information obtained through the five senses

B. Cause of a disease supported by medical data

C. Subjective information obtained through what the patient tells you

D. Actions for which the perioperative nurse is accountable

E. Any condition that requires a nursing intervention

F. Identification of a real or potential patient problem or risk

Additional Readings/Resources

Downing, D. (2009). The Perioperative Nursing Data Set. *AORN Journal, 89*(3), 600-602.

Battie', R.N. (2009). PNDS dashboard helps showcase Magnet accomplishments. *AORN Journal, 90*(2), 273-277.

Morton, P., Petersen, C., Chard, R., et al. (2013). Validation of the data elements for the health system domain of the PNDS. *AORN Journal, 98*(1), 39-48.

NANDA International, Inc. Retrieved Feb. 23, 2014, from http://www.nanda.org/

Petersen, C., & Kleiner, C. (2011). Evolution and revision of the Perioperative Nursing Data Set. *AORN Journal, 93*(1), 127-132.

Chapter Summary

The perioperative nurse's assessment of the surgical patient and formulation of nursing diagnoses are critical components of safe, efficient patient care. This information serves as the focal point for mapping the patient's perioperative experience.

Glossary

Advance directive — Legal document that allows the patient to provide instruction ahead of time on end-of-life care.

Age specific — Individual patient attributes based on stages of growth and development.

Allow natural death (AND) — Providing only comfort measures for the actively dying patient.

AORN standards and recommended practices — This term includes all sections of the *Perioperative Standards and Recommended Practices* published annually by AORN. The most current edition should be used at all times.

Assessment — Collecting data about a patient to determine the appropriate nursing diagnoses and expected outcomes. This includes patient's history and physical, vital signs, all aspects of presenting condition, and results of diagnostic tests. Assessment begins with data collection and ends with the formulation of nursing diagnoses. Assessment is ongoing during the perioperative period (i.e., includes preoperative, intraoperative, postoperative periods).

Association of periOperative Registered Nurses (AORN) — AORN is the professional organization of perioperative registered nurses that supports registered nurses in achieving optimal outcomes for patients undergoing operative and other invasive procedures. (www.aorn.org)

Community resources — Other agencies that the perioperative nurse may refer patients to for special needs (e.g., American Cancer Society, American Heart Association, home health care agencies, social services, organ procurement agencies).

Continuum of care — Care of patients undergoing operative or other invasive procedures from the time the decision to undergo surgery is made, through the intraoperative period, and for an undetermined postoperative period until the patient's health status is improved or a specified health goal is reached.

CPR directive — Provides for patient, agent, or guardian to refuse cardiopulmonary resuscitation.

Cultural diversity — Variances in beliefs, actions, customs, and values between racial, ethnic, religious, or social groups.

Discharge planning — The process of assessing the needs of patients for post-procedure care; developing a coordinated and multidisciplinary plan to provide the care required (including patient and family education, available services, and referral agencies and support groups); and evaluating the plan. The process begins before or on admission to the health care facility.

Documentation — The written record of nursing care including patient assessment, the actions taken as a result of that assessment, the plan of care developed and implemented, and the results of those actions. Documentation serves as the main, retrievable communication tool for the health care team.

Do-Not-Resuscitate (DNR) — Legal order written by a physician that respects a patient's request to not be resuscitated.

Family — For purposes of this guide, significant others and extended family are included in the term "family."

Health literacy — An integral part of patient education; the ability to read, understand, and follow instructions related to treatment.

Healthcare Insurance Portability and Accountability Act (HIPAA) — Legislation passed in 1996 that addresses various aspects of the use of patients' medical information, including confidentiality of patient information in the medical record, consent processes for access to patients' health information, and the right to sue the health plan provider.

Informed consent — The patient's right to make his or her own informed decisions based on information regarding treatment options, including the benefits, expected outcomes, risks, and potential complications; right to refuse treatment; and decisions regarding participation in research studies.

Interdisciplinary teams — Pharmacy, radiology, blood bank, laboratories, environmental services (i.e., housekeeping), biomedical engineering, etc.

Intervention (nursing) — Action taken based on patient assessment data with the intention of achieving one or more expected patient outcomes.

The Joint Commission — The independent accrediting organization that designates acceptable patient care and evaluates health care facilities' abilities to adhere to specific guidelines (e.g., documentation, processes, policies, and procedures). (www.jointcommission.org)

Living will — Document signed by patient refusing artificial life support measures in the event of terminal or irreversible illness.

Medical diagnosis — A disease-based determination of a condition by a physician based on a review of patient signs and symptoms and diagnostic tests.

Medical durable power of attorney — Designation of an agent to make health care decisions; it is not restricted to instances of terminal illness.

NANDA International, Inc. — The group that has developed a list of over 150 accepted nursing diagnoses to ensure that documentation in all areas of nursing uses consistent, comparable terminology. (www.nanda.org) Also see *Perioperative Nursing Data Set.*

Nursing diagnosis — A statement derived by the registered nurse from evaluating the patient's responses to actual or potential problems/conditions. The nursing diagnosis provides the framework for nursing interventions which, when implemented, will enable the patient to attain specific desired outcomes. It is structured using standardized nursing nomenclature. Also see North American Nursing Diagnosis Association and *Perioperative Nursing Data Set.*

Nursing process — The critical thinking a nurse uses to assess the health status of patients, identify problems, develop and implement plans of care, and evaluate the patients' responses to that care.

Outcome criteria — Statements developed to identify the tasks or conditions to be implemented that will assist the patient in achieving the desired outcomes. Outcome criteria indicate an expected, measurable change in the patient's health status.

Patient Self-Determination Act (PSDA) — The legal right to accept or refuse medical intervention, even if refusal will likely result in death.

Patients' rights — The rights of every patient to seek and receive health care regardless of his or her race, religion, or culture and with respect for the individual's self-image, privacy, and other such considerations, in accordance with the Patients' Bill of Rights.

Perioperative Nursing Data Set (PNDS) — The perioperative nursing vocabulary guidebook that provides nursing diagnosis, nursing interventions, and patient outcomes statements specific to the perioperative environment.

Perioperative period — Time commencing with the decision for surgical intervention and ending with a follow-up home/clinic evaluation. This period includes the preoperative, intraoperative, and postoperative phases.

Plan of care (or care plan) — A result of a systematic process of identifying expected patient outcomes and determining how to achieve them. It includes the list of interventions necessary to reach the expected outcome. The plan of care directs all nursing care activities related to each patient.

Postoperative phase — Begins with admission to the postanesthesia care area and ends with the resolution of surgical sequelae.

Preoperative phase — Begins when the decision for surgical intervention is made and ends with the transfer of the patient to the operating room bed.

Regulatory standards — Federal, state, and local laws and regulations that govern practice.

Safe environment — The setting in which the physical and psychological aspects of the environment are controlled for the purpose of presenting the least possible hazard to the patient, staff members, and community.

Surgical intervention — The patient's experiences during the preoperative, intraoperative, and postoperative phases, including the technical aspects and anatomical approach.

Surgical procedure — The technical aspects and anatomical approach used during surgical intervention.

Teaching and learning theories and techniques — Those aids and methods that facilitate learning (e.g., audiovisual tools, return demonstration, adult learning principles).

Time-out — As an integral component of The Joint Commission's Universal Protocol for Preventing Wrong Site, Wrong Procedure, and Wrong Person Surgery, a time-out surgical site verification must be conducted in the location where the procedure will be done, just before starting the procedure and, if possible, include active participation of the patient. It must involve the entire operative team, use active communication, be documented, and must include, at a minimum:
- Correct patient identity
- Correct side and site
- Agreement on the procedure to be done
- Correct patient position
- Availability of correct implants and any special equipment

References

AORN. (2011). *Perioperative Nursing Data Set* (3rd ed.). Denver: AORN, Inc.

AORN. (2014). *Perioperative Standards and Recommended Practices*. Denver: AORN, Inc.

Committee on Quality of Health Care in America, Institute of Medicine. (2001). *Cross-*

ing the Quality Chasm: A New Health System for the 21st Century. Washington, DC: National Academies Press.

Lewis, S.L., Dirksen, S.R., Heitkemper, M.M., et al. (2011). *Medical-Surgical Nursing: Assessment and Management of Clinical Problems* (8th ed.). St. Louis: Elsevier Mosby.

The Joint Commission. (2014). National Patient Safety Goals. Retrieved Feb. 23, 2014, from http://www.jointcommission.org/standards_information/npsgs.aspx

Rothrock, J.C. (Ed.). (2015). *Alexander's Care of the Patient in Surgery* (15th ed.). St. Louis: Mosby.

Swartz, M.H. (2010). *Textbook of Physical Diagnosis: History and Examination* (6th ed.). Philadelphia: Saunders Elsevier.

Answers to Chapter 1 Activities

Module 1: Assess the health status of the patient — Pages 37-41

Activity — Fill in the Blank

1. What sources of data will you utilize during Mr. J.'s assessment? *patient, family, the medical record, lab work, other health care providers, x-ray films, and diagnostic tests*

2. Which systems will be most important to assess during Mr. J.'s preoperative interview? *musculoskeletal, immune, GI, cardiovascular, integumentary*

Source: Rothrock, J. (2015). *Alexander's Care of the Patient in Surgery* (15th ed., pp. 3-5). St. Louis: Mosby.

Case Study Activity — Draw Your Own Concept Map

Make a list of all the data you feel you will need to address in your plan of care.

Assessment data to be used in development of plan of care:

- *Previous surgeries*
- *Elevated temperature (100° F, 37.8° C)*
- *Elevated WBCs*
- *Recent change in dentition*
- *Pain*
- *Age*
- *Heart block*
- *Current medications' influence on coagulation, healing*
- *Abnormal labs*
- *Heard of hearing*

From the patient information noted, begin drawing your concept map (at http://www.cc-institute. org/toolbox) that identifies the data you will need to use in developing your surgical plan of care. Put your patient's name, preoperative diagnosis, and proposed procedure in the center of the map.

See concept maps on pages 60-61 for answers to the following related questions.

- Identify Mr. J.'s "major problems," putting each into its own box.
- Arrange the data under their corresponding "major problems."

What critical information needs to be communicated to the following health care team members?

Anesthesia provider: ***History of GERD, hemoglobin/hematocrit lab values, history DVT, first degree heart block, temp, elevated WBCs, medical durable power of attorney***

Surgeon: ***Low-normal hemoglobin/hematocrit, history DVT, elevated temp and WBCs, medical durable power of attorney***

Scrub person: ***Availability of implants***

Case Study Activity — Critical Thinking

The following are common risk factors for infection. Based on your preoperative assessment of Mr. J., circle the items that put him at risk for a postoperative infection.

Nutritional status   dental health   age   existing infection (possible),   altered immune system

Source: Phillips, N. (2013). *Berry and Kohn's Operating Room Technique* (12th ed., pp. 117, 175).St. Louis: Mosby.

Activity — Matching

Match the patient assessment items on the left with the corresponding nursing intervention on the right. Note: Some items will have multiple answers. Answers may be used more than once.

Assessment Data:

Identification of patient: ***C, H***

Baseline vital signs (temperature, pulse, respirations, blood pressure, pulse oximetry reading, and pain assessment): ***E, F, I, J***

Height and weight: ***A, C, D, E, G***

Known medical conditions: ***A, B, C, D, E, F, G, I, J***

Prescription and over-the-counter medications, supplements including herbal preparations taken on a routine basis, and last medication administration: ***B, C, J***

Allergies or sensitivities, including latex and food: ***B, C, F, J***

NPO status: ***B, F***

Previous surgical history, including asking about metal implants and untoward reactions to anesthesia: ***A, B, C, D, E, F, G, H, I, J***

Skin condition: ***A, B, C, D, E, G, J***

Level of consciousness: ***B, D, F, H***

Emotional status: ***B, C, H***

Risk for falling: ***B, C, D***

Any history of drug or alcohol abuse: ***B, C, E***

Smoking history (packs per day and pack years): ***B, E, F***

Signs of physical or emotional abuse: ***B, G***

Diagnostic test results: ***A, B, C, E, F, G, J***

Diversity and cultural needs: ***B, H***

Knowledge deficits related to surgery/recovery: ***B, E, H***

Interventions:

A. Positioning

B. Patient education/ communication

C. Medication and solution administration

D. Moving/transfer

E. Infection prevention

F. Adequate airway/ oxygen exchange

G. Maintenance of skin integrity

H. Preventing wrong site, wrong patient, wrong procedure

I. Normothermia

J. Adequate tissue perfusion

> Source: Lewis, S.L., Dirksen, S.R., Heitkemper, M.M., et al. (2011). *Medical-Surgical Nursing: Assessment and Management of Clinical Problems.* St. Louis: Elsevier Mosby, pp. 335-344.

Activity — Critical Thinking

Read the following sentence, and then count the number of "f's" in the sentence. *Finished files are the result of years of scientific study combined with the experience of years.*

How many did you count? **_Six_** **_(Do not forget the "fs" in the words "of".)_**

> Source: Swartz, M.H. (2010). *Textbook of Physical Diagnosis: History and Examination* (6th ed.). Philadelphia: Saunders Elsevier, p. 129.

Module 2: Review of preoperative medications — Pages 42-43

Case Study Activity — Matching

Match Mr. J.'s current medications to the action from the list on the right:

Levothyroxine: ***D***

Ibuprofen: ***B***

Ginger: ***C***

Prednisone: ***A***

A. steroidal anti-inflammatory

B. nonsteroidal anti-inflammatory

C. complementary treatment for nausea, arthritis

D. suppresses TSH

> Source: epocrates online. Retrieved Feb. 23, 2014, from www.epocrates.com

Case Study Activity — Draw Your Own Concept Map, *continued*

SAMPLE Concept Map showing Mr. J.'s major problems.

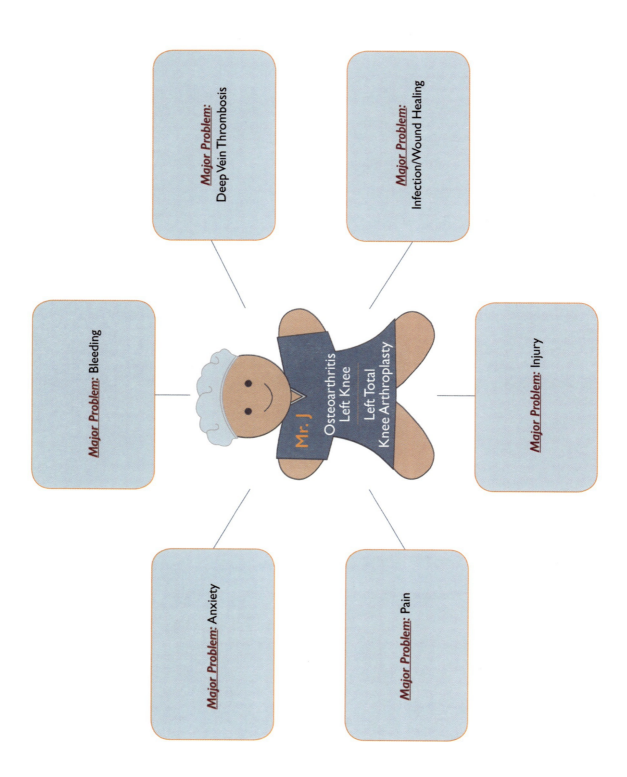

Case Study Activity — Draw Your Own Concept Map, *continued*

SAMPLE Concept Map showing the assessment data needed to develop a plan of care for Mr. J.

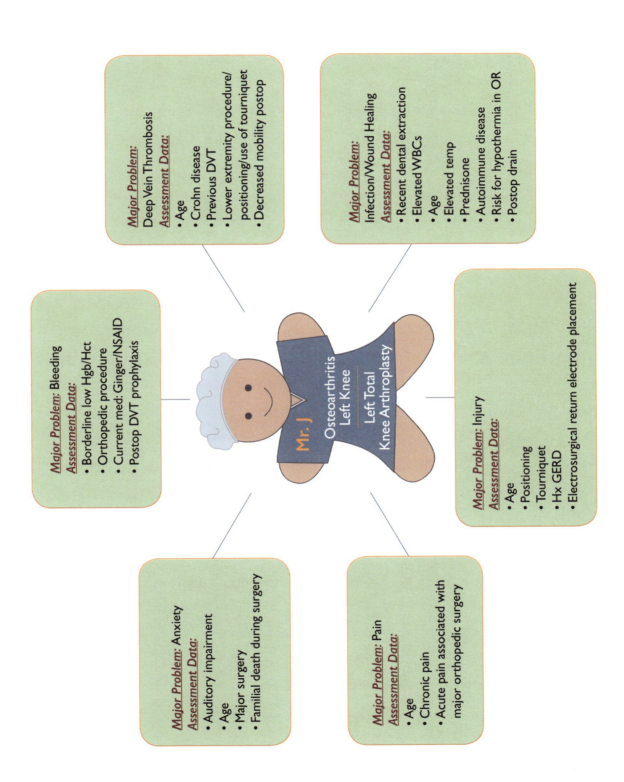

Major Problem: Deep Vein Thrombosis
Assessment Data:
- Age
- Crohn disease
- Previous DVT
- Lower extremity procedure/positioning/use of tourniquet
- Decreased mobility postop

Major Problem: Infection/Wound Healing
Assessment Data:
- Recent dental extraction
- Elevated WBCs
- Age
- Elevated temp
- Prednisone
- Autoimmune disease
- Risk for hypothermia in OR
- Postop drain

Major Problem: Bleeding
Assessment Data:
- Borderline low Hgb/Hct
- Orthopedic procedure
- Current med: Ginger/NSAID
- Postop DVT prophylaxis

Mr. J
Osteoarthritis Left Knee
Left Total Knee Arthroplasty

Major Problem: Injury
Assessment Data:
- Age
- Positioning
- Tourniquet
- Hx GERD
- Electrosurgical return electrode placement

Major Problem: Anxiety
Assessment Data:
- Auditory impairment
- Age
- Major surgery
- Familial death during surgery

Major Problem: Pain
Assessment Data:
- Age
- Chronic pain
- Acute pain associated with major orthopedic surgery

Case Study Activity — Critical Thinking

How will the use of a tourniquet during Mr. J.'s surgery affect the timing of the dose of his preoperative antibiotic?

Administration of the preoperative antibiotic may be adjusted to coordinate with the timing of the tourniquet to promote optimal drug perfusion of the incision site.

> Source: AORN. (2014). Recommended practices: Pneumatic tourniquet. In *Perioperative Standards and Recommended Practices,* p. 188.. Denver: AORN, Inc.

Which of Mr. J.'s medications could influence the surgical procedure? Why?

Ibuprofen increases bleeding time; Prednisone can prolong healing time. In addition, Mr. J.'s use of ginger may increase the anticoagulant effect of warfarin if he is placed on it postoperatively.

> Sources: Rothrock, J. (2015). *Alexander's Care of the Patient in Surgery* (15th ed., p. 1169). St. Louis: Mosby; epocrates online. Retrieved Feb. 23, 2014, from www.epocrates.com

Module 3: Initiation of the Universal Protocol — Pages 43-45

Activity — Fill in the Blank

What three "wrongs" will implementation of the Universal Protocol help prevent?

Patient   Site   Procedure

> Source: Rothrock, J. (2015). *Alexander's Care of the Patient in Surgery* (15th ed., p. 24). St. Louis: Mosby.

Activity — Critical Thinking

Identify the corresponding AORN standard or recommended practice that addresses each of the following "never events."

1. Surgery performed on the wrong body part, the wrong patient, or the wrong procedure
   Position statement on preventing wrong-patient, wrong-site, wrong-procedure events

2. Unintended retention of a foreign object in a patient after surgery or other procedure
   Recommended practices: Prevention of retained surgical items

3. Patient death or serious disability associated with a medication error
   Recommended practices: Medication safety

4. Patient death or serious disability associated with a burn incurred from any source
   Recommended practices: Laser safety, Electrosurgery, Preoperative patient skin antisepsis

5. Hospital acquired pressure ulcer
   Recommended practices: Positioning the patient

6. Deep vein thrombosis
   Recommended practices: Prevention of deep vein thrombosis

7. Hospital acquired surgical site infections
   Recommended practices: Surgical attire, Hand hygiene, Sterile technique, Traffic patterns, Environmental cleaning, Prevention of transmissible infections, Prevention of hypothermia, Preoperative patient skin antisepsis, Sterilization

   Source: AORN. (2014). *Perioperative Standards and Recommended Practices*. Denver: AORN, Inc.

Activity — Mark the Site

Mark the illustration to correspond with the correct site and side for Mr. J.'s surgery.

A line, initials, or "yes" are all acceptable, and should be drawn on the left thigh. Marking should be visible after Mr. J. has been prepped and draped.

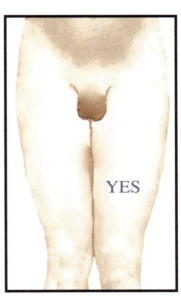

   Source: Rothrock, J. (2015). *Alexander's Care of the Patient in Surgery* (15th ed., p. 29). St. Louis: Mosby.

Module 4: Obtaining surgical consent — Pages 45-47

Activity — Fill in the Blank

The surgeon or practitioner performing the procedure is responsible for informing the patient about the proposed procedure in terms that he or she can understand.

It is the ***surgeon's or practitioner's*** responsibility to obtain informed consent.

   Source: Rothrock, J. (2015). *Alexander's Care of the Patient in Surgery* (15th ed., pp. 42, 44). St. Louis: Mosby.

Activity — Critical Thinking

How does obtaining surgical consent for a child differ from that of an adult?

The person legally responsible for the child, rather than the patient, agrees to the procedure after being informed of the risks, benefits, and alternatives of the proposed procedure. Unless emancipated, a child under the age of 18 cannot sign his/her own consent. Children should be included in the discussion, and preoperative teaching should take into account age-specific needs and the extent the patient is able to understand and participate in the decision-making

process. Both legal guardian and patient should have the opportunity to have questions answered.

Source: Rothrock, J. (2015). *Alexander's Care or the Patient in Surgery* (15th ed., pp. 1011-1012). St. Louis: Mosby.

Case Study Activity — Consent

Mr. J.'s consent and the surgery schedule read right total knee arthroplasty. Mr. J., the H&P, and knee films all state that the left knee is the correct operative site. How will you address this discrepancy?

The discrepancy between the consent, patient expectations, and other documents should be brought to the attention of the surgeon. The surgery schedule should be corrected, and other members of Mr. J.'s health care team notified. The consent (if paper) should be corrected by drawing a line through the incorrect information with the date, time, and initials of the surgeon and Mr. J.

Source: Phillips, N. (2013). *Berry and Kohn's Operating Room Technique* (12th ed., p. 48). St. Louis: Mosby. .

Module 5: Ensuring patients' rights by providing information on advance directives, do-not-resuscitate — Pages 47-49

Activity — True or False

Under the Patient Self-Determination Act, patients have the legal right to accept or refuse medical treatment, including resuscitation, even if refusal will likely result in death.

True: Under the Patient Self-Determination Act, patients have the legal right to accept or refuse medical treatment, including resuscitation, even if refusal will likely result in death.

Source: Rothrock, J. (2015). *Alexander's Care of the Patient in Surgery* (15th ed., p. 44). St. Louis: Mosby.

Mr. J. has brought his completed medical durable power of attorney form with him. It states that he does not wish life-sustaining measures for an irreversible condition. He says, "I guess I won't be needing this during my surgery." What is your response?

Sample response:
"It is important to have your wishes respected throughout your entire surgical experience. Let's include your anesthesia care provider, surgeon, and your family members in this discussion so that we all understand the implications of the decision made."

Source: AORN. (2014). Exhibit B: Perioperative explications. In *Perioperative Standards and Recommended Practices*, p. 24. Denver: AORN, Inc.; Rothrock, J.C. (2015). *Alexander's Care of the Patient in Surgery* (15th ed., pp. 44, 1102). St. Louis: Mosby.

Module 6: Pain assessment — Pages 49-50

Activity — Matching

Match the most appropriate pain rating scale to the patient identified below (answers may be used more than once)

3-year-old: **B**

45-year-old man: **A, C**

23-year-old woman who does not speak English: **B**

A. 0-10 Numeric pain intensity scale

B. FACES Pain rating scale

C. Simple descriptive pain intensity scale

> Source: Rothrock, J. (2015). *Alexander's Care of the Patient in Surgery* (15th ed., p. 282). St. Louis: Mosby.

Case Study Activity — Pain Assessment

While discussing Mr. J.'s pain management plan, he tells you, "I don't plan on taking any of that stuff; I don't want to get addicted." What is your response?

"The treatment of acute postoperative pain is different from the chronic abuse of narcotics. Managing your pain will actually help you recover more quickly. Providing pain medication during your surgery via an epidural catheter may decrease the amount of general anesthetic you'll need. Using a patient controlled anesthesia pump postoperatively will allow you to determine when you get your pain medicine. You'll be able to get out of bed and walk sooner, and be able to get the most benefit from your physical therapy exercises. Let's talk with your anesthesia care provider about the best options for you."

> Source: Rothrock, J. (2015). *Alexander's Care of the Patient in Surgery* (15th ed., pp. 280-286). St. Louis: Mosby.

Module 7: Development of nursing diagnoses — Pages 51-52

Activity — Matching

Match the term to its correct definition:

Etiology: **B**

Nursing diagnosis: **F**

Nursing intervention: **D**

Problem: **E**

Sign: **A**

Symptom: **C**

A. Objective information obtained through the five senses

B. Cause of a disease supported by medical data

C. Subjective information obtained through what the patient tells you

D. Actions for which the perioperative nurse is accountable

E. Any condition that requires a nursing intervention

F. Identification of a real or potential patient problem or risk

Source: Venes, D. (ed.). (2013). *Tabor's Cyclopedic Medical Dictionary.* Philadelphia, PA: F.A. Davis Co.

Case Study Activity — Nursing Diagnoses

From your interpretation of Mr. J.'s assessment data, formulate nursing diagnoses to address each identified problem or potential problem. Write your nursing diagnoses in the boxes next to your "major problem" in your concept map in the Study Guide Toolbox at http://www.cc-institute.org/toolbox. Not all of your "major problems" may have a corresponding nursing diagnosis. ***Sample answers added to the map below.***

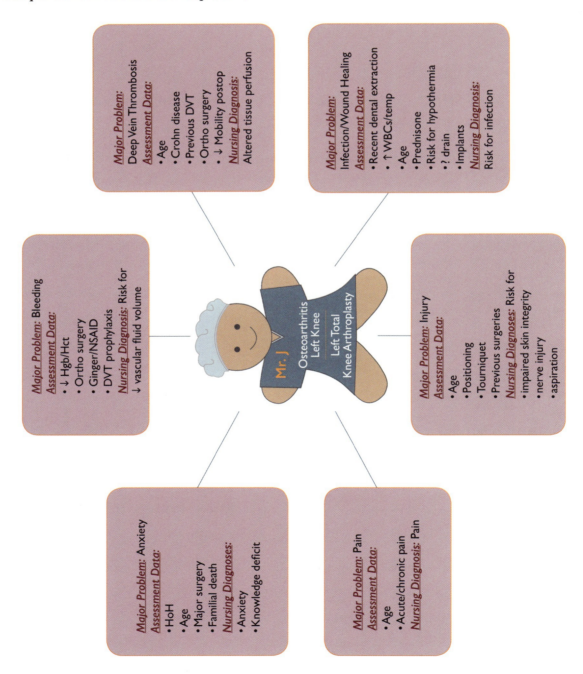

CHAPTER 2:
Identify Expected Outcomes and Develop an Individualized Plan of Care

Test Specifications:
9% of CNOR test questions are based on Identify Expected Outcomes and Develop an Individualized Plan of Care.

Introduction

Perioperative nurses use critical thinking and clinical judgment to set priorities and identify the desirable outcomes of patient care.

The plan of care is derived from nursing diagnoses and is developed through effective communication with the patient and other parties as appropriate. The plan should be patient centered, be culturally considerate, and provide for continuity of care. After all, the intraoperative experience is just one event in the patient's life. Encouraging the patient to take an active role in the overall plan preserves his or her autonomy, privacy, dignity, and rights.

Organizing the components of patient care can be confusing, so different methods have been developed to categorize and define nursing terminology and actions. The *Perioperative Nursing Data Set* (PNDS) is a standardized language that has incorporated perioperative nursing diagnoses, interventions, and outcomes (AORN, 2011). The PNDS will be used throughout this chapter as the template for the development of care plans. It is not the only taxonomy used in the nursing profession, but it is specific to the perioperative arena. Many electronic medical records have incorporated the PNDS into their charting systems. The glossary in this chapter includes definitions for the terms used in the PNDS, and frequently used nursing diagnoses are provided in Chapter 1 on page 51.

This chapter provides opportunities to identify expected outcomes and develop plans of care for the surgical patient based on your assessment. Measurable patient data are used to develop specific outcomes. Suggestions for individualizing the plan of care are provided. For the purposes of this chapter, we will continue to build on the information captured in the concept map begun in Chapter 1 (page 39) in the Toolbox at http://www.cc-institute/toolbox

Module 1: Develop Measurable Patient Outcomes from Patient Assessment Data and Nursing Diagnoses

Outcomes can be considered the goals or desired end results of nursing, or "nurse sensitive" interventions. In the case of perioperative nursing, they are what we want our patients to be able to do or exhibit at the end of a procedure. By developing expected outcomes, the perioperative nurse is able to:

1. Select appropriate nursing interventions to be used in the plan of care.
2. Determine a baseline against which to measure success of the intervention.
3. Identify reasonable time frames in which to achieve goals.

Outcomes should be realistic, culturally sensitive, age-specific, and written in measurable terms. Interdisciplinary collaboration and patient expectations are equally important in helping to identify the best outcomes for the patient based on available resources.

Competency Outcomes

To successfully complete the activities in this module, you will need to be able to:

1. Construct perioperative patient outcome statements based on assessment data and nursing diagnoses.
2. List three advantages of developing patient outcomes that can be included in a plan of care.

Recommended Readings

Alexander's Care of the Patient in Surgery. (2015, 15th ed.), Chapter 1: Concepts basic to perioperative nursing; Unit II: Surgical interventions.

Berry and Kohn's Operating Room Technique. (2013, 12th ed.), Chapter 2: Foundations of perioperative patient care standards.

Perioperative Standards and Recommended Practices. (2014), Section II: Recommended practices for perioperative nursing; Section III: Guidance statements.

Key Words

Measurable, nurse sensitive, nursing intervention, outcome, PNDS

Activity — Short Answer

Three benefits of identifying expected outcomes are that the perioperative nurse will be able to:

1.

2.

3.

> **"Go To"**
> **Case Study Activity**
>
> For the concept map you have developed in the Toolbox (at http://www.cc-institute.org/toolbox) add patient outcomes to the appropriate boxes.

Additional Readings/Resources

Lamberg, E., Salantera, S., & Junttila, K. (2013). Evaluating perioperative nursing in Finland: An initial validation of Perioperative Nursing Data Set outcomes. *AORN Journal, 98*(2), 172-185.

Module 2: Develop an Individualized Plan of Care

Plans of care are developed using the information obtained during the patient assessment and corresponding nursing diagnoses. The perioperative registered nurse must prioritize patient problems, work within a multidisciplinary environment, develop criteria for evaluation, and utilize evidence-based practice — in the five minutes taken to interview and assess the patient! The plan shapes the course of care for the patient, and for that reason, it should be based on the most current best practices. It should be easily understood and accessed by all health care providers; therefore, clear, comprehensive documentation of nursing interventions is needed to validate nursing practice and patient outcomes.

Caring for patients across the lifespan requires that the perioperative nurse applies the nursing process to meet the age-specific needs of the patient. Various theories address psychosocial, sensory, and aging-associated phases of human growth and development (Rothrock, 2015, p. 1009). Regardless of a patient's age, the perioperative nurse develops a care plan that is directed toward avoiding or resolving patient problems.

Competency Outcomes

To successfully complete the activities in this module, you will need to be able to:

1. Develop an individualized plan of care that addresses the patient's potential physiologic and psychosocial responses to the surgical experience.
2. Collaborate with the interdisciplinary health care team to address identified risks (e.g., injury from positioning, infection, hypothermia).

Recommended Readings

Alexander's Care of the Patient in Surgery. (2015, 15th ed.), Chapter 1: Concepts basic to perioperative nursing; Unit II: Surgical interventions.

Berry and Kohn's Operating Room Technique. (2013, 12th ed.), Chapter 2: Foundations of perioperative patient care standards; Chapter 7: The patient: The reason for your existence; Chapter 9: Perioperative geriatrics; Chapter 11: Ambulatory surgery centers and alternative surgical locations; Chapter 21: Preoperative preparation of the patient.

Perioperative Standards and Recommended Practices. (2014), Section 1: Standards of perioperative nursing; Section II: Recommended practices for perioperative nursing; Section III: Guidance statements.

Key Words

Age-specific, nursing diagnosis, nursing interventions, nursing process, patient problems, plan of care

Activity — Fill in the Blank

Fill in the patient outcome and nursing interventions for each of the following scenarios:

1. Nursing diagnosis: Knowledge deficit related to procedure
    Assessment data:
    Objective: Patient is scheduled for laparoscopic bilateral tubal ligation.
    Subjective: Patient states: "I'll be so happy when I don't have such terrible cramps with my periods anymore. Maybe this means I'll be able to get pregnant now."

    Patient outcome: _____

    Nursing interventions: _____

2. Nursing diagnosis: Risk for infection
    Assessment data:
    Objective: Patient is scheduled for ventral hernia repair with mesh. She is on long-term corticosteroids for the treatment of systemic lupus erythrematosis (SLE). Assessment of skin integrity shows multiple areas of bruising on arms and legs.
    Subjective: "My skin is like tissue paper, and I take forever to heal, even when it's just a small cut or scrape."

    Patient outcome: _____

    Nursing interventions: _____

3. Nursing diagnosis: Risk for developing hypothermia
    Assessment data:
    Objective: 3-month-old boy scheduled for cleft lip repair. Patient's temperature (temporal artery) is 37.2° C.

    Patient outcome: _____

    Nursing interventions: _____

4. Nursing diagnosis: Risk for perioperative positioning injury
    Assessment data:
    Objective: Patient is scheduled for transurethral resection of the prostate (TURP). Subjective: "I feel like the bionic man. I've had both hips replaced."

    Patient outcome: _____

    Nursing interventions: _____

Additional Readings/Resources

Bashaw, M., & Scott, D.N. (2012). Surgical risk factors in geriatric perioperative patients. *AORN Journal, 96*(1), 58-74.

Doerflinger, D.M.C. (2009). Older adult surgical patients: Presentation and challenges. *AORN Journal, 90*(2), 223-242. Bonus: Examination questions follow the article.

Tonge, A. (2011). Perioperative care of the pediatric patient with Down syndrome. *AORN Journal, 94*(6), 606-617.

"Go To" Case Study Activity

For each box in your concept map in the Toolbox at http://www.cc-institute.org/toolbox, list the nursing interventions needed to meet the identified outcomes/goals.

Module 3: Incorporate Patient Education Into the Plan of Care

Teaching is an essential role of the professional nurse. Assessing the patient's readiness to learn, identifying barriers to learning, and establishing prior knowledge of the event provide a preliminary framework from which the nurse establishes a teaching-learning plan specific to the patient's needs. The perioperative nurse acts as the patient advocate and practices according to the *ANA Code of Ethics for Nurses* (AORN, 2014).

As individuals, patients experience a range of responses to the surgical experience. Many variables affect an individual's ability to learn — the type of surgery, reason for surgery, available resources and support services, age of the patient, and cultural and spiritual needs. Surgery is a stressful event, and it affects the patient's ability to hear and process information.

Facilities must comply with The Joint Commission regulations on patient education in order to be accredited, but teaching our patients goes beyond legal requirements. Patients who understand their treatment plan are less likely to be readmitted or have infections or other complications. A knowledgeable patient is one of the most cost-effective goals a facility can strive to achieve.

The immediate preoperative setting, however, is not an ideal environment for patient education. Anxiety, time constraints, and preoperative medications do not provide an atmosphere conducive to learning new materials or retaining information.

The perioperative nurse is wise to prioritize and limit teaching strategies to:

1. What does the patient already know?
2. What does the patient need to know?
3. What factors will enhance or inhibit the learning experience?
4. What is the best method for sharing information?
5. How will I know that the patient understands what has been taught?

Competency Outcomes

To successfully complete the activities in this module, you will need to be able to:

1. Incorporate patient rights and responsibilities into a teaching plan.
2. Recognize the impact of surgical stressors (medications, pain, and anxiety) on the ability to learn.
3. Identify community and institutional resources based on identified patient needs.
4. Incorporate The Joint Commission's requirements for patient education into a teaching plan.
5. Identify barriers and aids to learning.

Recommended Readings

Alexander's Care of the Patient in Surgery. (2015, 15th ed.), Unit II: Surgical interventions; Unit III: Special considerations.

Berry and Kohn's Operating Room Technique. (2013, 12th ed.), Chapter 2: Foundations of perioperative patient care standards; Chapter 21: Preoperative preparation of the patient.

Perioperative Standards and Recommended Practices. (2014), Exhibit B: Perioperative explications for the ANA Code of Ethics for Nurses, pp. 21-42.

Key Words

Age-specific, barriers, patient education, teach back

Case Study Activity

1. How can you determine what Mr. J. already knows about his upcoming surgery?

2. What does Mr. J. need to know to participate in his plan of care?

3. What are Mr. J.'s strengths/barriers to learning?

4. How can you determine that Mr. J. understands what you have told him?

5. What resources can you recommend to assist Mr. J. postoperatively with the problems you've identified? How will he access these resources?

"Go To" Activity — Skill Building

Serve as a resource for a preoperative patient education class.

Additional Readings/Resources:

AMA Health Literacy Resources. (2014). Retrieved Feb. 26, 2014, from http://www. ama-assn.org/ama/pub/about-ama/ama-foundation/our-programs/public-health/health-literacy-program/health-literacy-kit.page
Note: Toolkit costs $35 but comes with an excellent video, which is worth the cost.

Bailey, L. (2010). Strategies for decreasing patient anxiety in the perioperative setting. *AORN Journal, 92*(4), 445-460.

Byrne, M.M. (2011). Information literacy: Implications for perioperative nurses. *AORN Journal, 93*(2), 282-286.

Kruzik, N. (2009). Benefits of preoperative education for adult elective surgery patients. *AORN Journal, 90*(3), 381-387.

Ortoleva, C. (2010). An approach to consistent patient education. *AORN Journal, 92*(4), 437-444.

Pashley, H.S. (2012). Overcoming barriers when caring for patients with limited English proficiency. *AORN Journal, 96*(3), C10-C11.

Petersen, C., & Kleiner, C. (2011). Evolution and revision of the Perioperative Nursing Data Set. *AORN Journal, 93*(1), 127-132.

Sayin, Y., & Aksoy, G. (2012). The nurse's role in providing information to surgical patients and family members in Turkey: A descriptive study. *AORN Journal, 95*(6), 772-787.

Sorenson, H.L., Card, C.A., Malley, M.T., & Strzelecki, J. M. (2009). Using a collaborative child life approach for continuous surgical preparation. *AORN Journal, 90*(4), 557-566.

Chapter Summary

Managing the care of perioperative patients requires critical thinking, independent judgment in clinical decision making, collaboration among all other health care professionals, and an ethical code to guide practice. By using the nursing process, the perioperative nurse prioritizes patient problems identified by objective and subjective data.

Patient centered outcomes are determined from the nursing diagnoses and are written in measurable terms. Nursing interventions are designed to achieve the established outcomes, and through evaluation, the outcomes may be renegotiated and revised.

The examples found throughout this chapter reflect perioperative patient outcomes, outcome definitions, and outcome indicators. Note that the indicators are observable and measurable. The goal for the development of a plan of care is to identify and address the needs of the patient through the provision of quality, evidence-based practice.

Glossary

Age specific — Patient characteristics based on stages of growth and development.

Family — For purposes of this guide, significant others and extended family are included in the term "family."

Health care team — The providers of patient care services who are required to provide direct patient care to help the patient achieve a positive outcome. Support services include but are not limited to pharmacy, radiology, blood bank, housekeeping, etc.

NANDA International, Inc. — The group that has developed a list of over 150 accepted nursing diagnoses to ensure that documentation in all areas of nursing use consistent, comparable terminology. (www.nanda.org) Also see *Perioperative Nursing Data Set.*

Nursing diagnosis — A statement derived from the nursing assessment data that provides the framework for nursing interventions that enable the patient to attain specific desired outcomes. It is structured using standardized nursing nomenclature. Also see North American Nursing Diagnosis Association and *Perioperative Nursing Data Set.*

Nursing intervention — Actions initiated by the nurse to assist the patient in reaching a desired outcome.

Nursing process — The critical thinking a nurse uses to assess the health status of patients, identify problems, develop and implement plans of care, and evaluate the patients' responses to that care.

Perioperative Nursing Data Set (PNDS) — The perioperative nursing vocabulary guidebook that provides nursing diagnosis, nursing interventions, and patient outcomes statements specific to the perioperative environment.

Terms specific to the PNDS:

Domain — The four overall divisions of the conceptual framework of the *Perioperative Nursing Data Set.* All interventions and expected outcomes relate to one or more domains. The four domains are Safety, Physiologic Responses, Behavioral Responses, and the Health System.

Outcome — Outcomes are designed to direct and evaluate patient care and are part of the overall plan of care. The perioperative nurse in collaboration with the patient formulates the outcomes from the nursing diagnoses. In the case of the PNDS, the outcomes serve as positive statements reflecting expected achievement of identified goals (AORN, 2011). Outcomes should be written in a concise, measurable, and realistic manner. Documentation of the plan of care, expected outcomes, and nursing interventions provides a means for evaluation.

Outcome indicator — Measures of performance that link nursing interventions to outcomes. Typically, an indicator is a clinical finding, although it may be an administrative quality benchmark (as in documentation) or a fiscal value (as in cost-effective measures).

Applicable nursing diagnosis — A statement derived from the nursing assessment data that provides the framework for nursing interventions. The diagnosis may be a real or potential problem. It is structured using standardized nursing terms.

Intervention — An action taken based on patient assessment data with the intention of achieving one or more expected patient outcomes.

Evaluation — The final step in the nursing process in which success of interventions in meeting outcomes is measured.

Plan of care (or care plan) — A result of a systematic process of identifying expected patient outcomes and determining how to achieve them. It includes the list of interventions necessary to reach the expected outcome. The plan of care directs all nursing care activities related to each patient.

Support services — Pharmacy, radiology, blood bank, laboratories, environmental services (i.e., housekeeping), biomedical engineering, etc.

Teach back — A method of assessing the effectiveness of patient education by asking the patient to repeat, or "teach back," important components of the instruction.

Transfer — Moving a patient from one place to another (e.g., to or from a bed or stretcher).

Transport — Moving a patient via a device (e.g., wheelchair, stretcher, wagon).

References

AORN. (2011). *Perioperative Nursing Data Set* (3rd ed.). Denver: AORN, Inc.

AORN. (2014). Exhibit B: Perioperative explications for the ANA Code of Ethics for nurses. In *Perioperative Standards and Recommended Practices*. Denver: AORN, Inc.

Phillips, N. (2013). *Berry and Kohn's Operating Room Technique* (12th ed.). St. Louis: Mosby.

Rothrock, J.C. (Ed.). (2015). *Alexander's Care of the Patient in Surgery* (15th ed.). St. Louis: Mosby.

Answers to Chapter 2 Activities

Module 1: Develop measurable patient outcomes from patient assessment data and nursing diagnoses — Pages 68-69

Activity — Short Answer

Three benefits of identifying expected outcomes are that the perioperative nurse will be able to:
1. *Select appropriate nursing interventions to be used in the plan of care.*
2. *Determine a baseline against which to measure success of the intervention.*
3. *Identify realistic time frames in which to achieve goals.*

> Sources: Phillips, N. (2013). *Berry and Kohn Operating Room Technique* (12th ed., pp. 32-33). St. Louis: Mosby. Rothrock, J. (2015). *Alexander's Care of the Patient in Surgery* (15th ed., pp. 5-6). St. Louis: Mosby.

"Go To" Case Study Activity

From the concept map you have developed on the CD for Mr. J., add patient outcomes to the appropriate boxes. *Examples are provided on the next page, but are not to be considered all-inclusive.*

> Sources: Rothrock, J. (2015). *Alexander's Care of the Patient in Surgery* (15th ed., p. 5). St. Louis: Mosby. AORN. (2014). *Perioperative Standards and Recommended Practices,* Sections II and III. Denver: AORN, Inc.

Module 2: Develop an individualized plan of care — Pages 69-71

Activity — Fill in the Blank

Fill in the patient outcome and nursing interventions for each of the following scenarios. *Examples are provided below, but are not to be considered all-inclusive.*

1. Nursing diagnosis: Knowledge deficit related to procedure
   Assessment data:
       Objective: Patient is scheduled for laparoscopic bilateral tubal ligation.
       Subjective: Patient states: "I'll be so happy when I don't have such terrible cramps with my periods anymore. Maybe this means I'll be able to get pregnant now."

   Patient outcome: Patient demonstrates knowledge of physiologic responses to surgical procedure.
   Nursing interventions: Implement the Universal Protocol (correct patient, correct surgery, correct site). Confirm stated procedure with schedule and consent. Notify surgeon of discrepancy between patient's understanding of procedure and scheduled surgery.

"Go To" Case Study Activity

SAMPLE Concept map listing the nursing interventions needed to meet the identified outcomes.

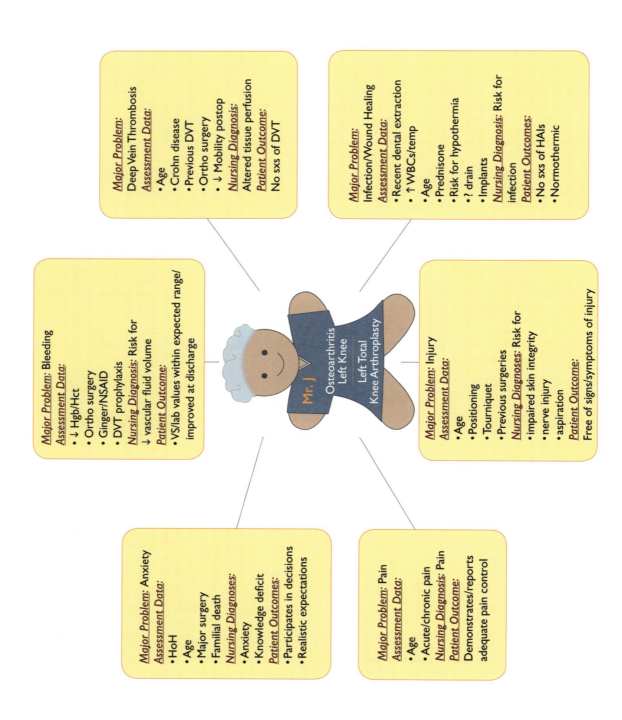

2. Nursing diagnosis: Risk for infection
   Assessment data:
   > Objective: Patient is scheduled for ventral hernia repair with mesh. She is on long-term corticosteroids for the treatment of systemic lupus erythrematosis (SLE). Assessment of skin integrity shows multiple areas of bruising on arms and legs.
   > Subjective: "My skin is like tissue paper, and I take forever to heal, even when it's just a small cut or scrape."

   Patient outcome: The patient is free of signs and symptoms of infection.
   Nursing interventions: Implement and maintain aseptic technique; implement protective measures to prevent injury to skin.

3. Nursing diagnosis: Risk for developing hypothermia
   Assessment data:
   > Objective: 3-month-old boy scheduled for cleft lip repair. Patient's temperature (temporal artery) is 37.2° C.

   Patient outcome: Patient is at or returning to normothermia at conclusion of procedure.
   Nursing interventions: Limit skin exposure to operative site; implement thermoregulation measures (prewarming, warming devices, warm IV fluids, increase room temperature, provide equipment for anesthesia provider to humidify/warm anesthetic gases). Use a reliable site for measuring core temperature.

4. Nursing diagnosis: Risk for perioperative positioning injury
   Assessment data:
   > Objective: Patient is scheduled for transurethral resection of the prostate (TURP).
   > Subjective: "I feel like the bionic man. I've had both hips replaced."

   Patient outcome: Patient is free of signs and symptoms of injury related to positioning; regains normal mobility postoperatively.
   Nursing interventions: Obtain positioning aids and padding. Avoid hyperabduction of hips/leaning on inner thighs. Avoid high stirrups and use boot stirrups if possible. Position stirrups at the same height and ensure that devices are securely attached to OR bed. Limit time in lithotomy position by efficient use of OR time and resources. Legs should be lifted and removed from stirrups slowly and simultaneously; return legs to bed one at a time if possible. Evaluate for signs and symptoms of injury related to positioning.

Sources: AORN. (2014). Recommended practices: Sterile technique; Positioning the patient in the perioperative practice setting; Prevention of hypothermia. In *Perioperative Standards and Recommended Practices.* Denver: AORN, Inc. Rothrock, J.C. (Ed.). (2015, pp. 3, 5, 7). *Alexander's Care of the Patient in Surgery* (15th ed.). St. Louis: Mosby.

"Go To" Case Study Activity

For each box in your concept map on the CD, list the nursing interventions needed to meet the identified outcomes/goals. ***Examples are provided on the following page, but are not to be considered all-inclusive.***

"Go To" Case Study Activity

SAMPLE Concept map listing the nursing interventions needed to meet the identified outcomes/goals.

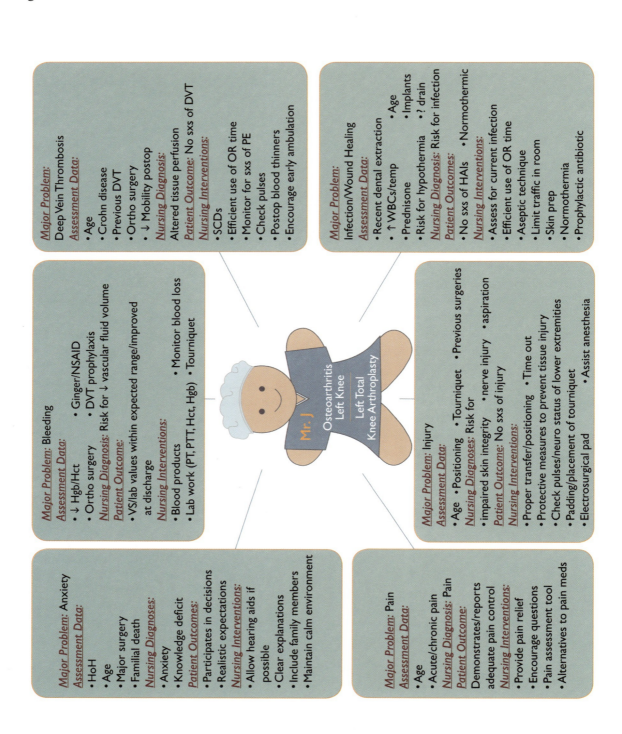

Module 3: Incorporate patient education into the plan of care — Pages 71-74

Case Study Activity

1. How can you determine what Mr. J. already knows about his upcoming surgery?

Ask Mr. J. to describe in his own words his planned surgery, the reason(s) for it, and the proposed plan of care (length of stay, type of anesthesia, rehabilitation, restrictions on activity, expectations related to pain management, etc.).

2. What does Mr. J. need to know to participate in his plan of care?

Mr. J. needs to be provided information on the perioperative plan of care in terms that he understands. Adequate time needs to be provided to answer his and his family's questions. Information needs to be prioritized so that the most important information (surgery and immediate postoperative period) are covered.

3. What are Mr. J.'s strengths/barriers to learning?

Strengths:
    Well educated
    Values independence

Barriers:
    Unfamiliar learning environment (hospital)
    No immediate support person at home
    Hard of hearing

Source: Rothrock, J. (2015, pp. 698; 1098-1099). *Alexander's Care of the Patient in Surgery* (15th ed.). St. Louis: Mosby.

4. How can you determine that Mr. J. understands what you have told him?

By having him teach back or demonstrate back (as appropriate) the information he has received.

Source: Phillips, N. (2013, pp. 377-378). *Berry and Kohn's Operating Room Technique*. St. Louis: Mosby.

5. What resources can you recommend to assist Mr. J. postoperatively with the problems you've identified? How will he access these resources?

* Note: the following references are examples only; CCI does not endorse any of these programs or organizations. Web site addresses were accurate as of Feb. 26, 2014.

Hospital-based wellness classes: Check with your facility's case manager for a list of resources that are available both in-house and in the community.

Home care after discharge:
Visiting Nurse Association or other organization to assist with ADL's as needed when discharged to home.
http://www.thevnacares.org/

Crohn's support group:
Crohn's and Colitis Foundation of America
http://www.ccfa.org/living-with-crohns-colitis/find-a-support-group/

Nutritional resources: National Agricultural Library, USDA http://www.nutrition.gov/lifestages/seniors

CHAPTER 3:
Intraoperative Activities

> **Test Specifications:**
> *31% of CNOR test questions are based on Intraoperative Activities.*

Introduction

The intraoperative phase begins when the patient enters the operating room (OR) or procedure area and ends when the patient is transferred to the postanesthesia care unit (PACU), intensive care unit (ICU), or other level of care. During this phase, the patient receives anesthetic agents; is positioned, prepped, and draped; and undergoes the operative or invasive procedure. The practice of perioperative nursing requires a combination of active assessment, collaboration, technical skills, and critical thinking skills unique to this area of nursing.

As one member of a multidisciplinary team who focuses solely on the surgical patient's needs, the perioperative RN serves as the primary patient advocate while coordinating the efforts of all team members toward the goal of optimal patient outcomes. This already Herculean task is compounded by today's ever-expanding arsenal of new technology including robotics, remote surgeries, novel applications of minimally invasive procedures, and "biologic" implant and graft materials. Our patients are sicker, our time spent with them is shorter, and both the consumer and the facility demand quality, efficient, cost-effective health care experiences. Today's perioperative RN is challenged to continually update an existing knowledge base through lifelong learning and ongoing education.

This chapter will help you review the competencies needed to safely care for the patient in the intraoperative phase of surgery. The plan of care developed for our patient in Chapters 1 and 2 will be incorporated into intraoperative nursing interventions. Concepts including maintenance of aseptic technique, risk factors for environmental injury, emotional and sociocultural issues, and health system and regulatory standards, regulation, and guidelines are applied to clinical learning activities.

Module 1: Introduction of the Patient to the Operative/Procedure Area

Every patient has unique physical and behavioral responses to stresses encountered during the surgical procedure, regardless of the setting. These responses must be taken into account as the perioperative nurse incorporates appropriate nursing interventions and evaluates their effectiveness. The first task when the patient enters the operative or procedure area is to provide a safe environment that is supportive of not only a patient's physiologic needs, but also his/her beliefs, personal rights, and dignity.

Competency Outcomes

To successfully complete the activities in this module, you will need to be able to:

1. Appraise behavioral responses of the patient and family to the surgical experience.
2. Review components of the time-out.
3. Design activities to address common physiologic responses to the surgical experience.
4. Apply measures to promote patient comfort and safety.

Recommended Readings

Alexander's Care of the Patient in Surgery. (2015, 15th ed.), Chapter 2: Patient safety and risk management; Chapter 4: Infection prevention and control in the perioperative setting; Chapter 6: Positioning the patient for surgery.

Berry and Kohn's Operating Room Technique. (2013, 12th ed.), Chapter 2: Foundations of perioperative patient care standards; Chapter 7: The patient: The reason for your existence; Chapter 11: Ambulatory surgery centers and alternative surgical locations; Chapter 21: Preoperative preparation of the patient; Chapter 25: Coordinated roles of the scrub person and the circulating nurse.

Perioperative Standards and Recommended Practices. (2014), Guidance statement:
• Safe patient handling and movement.

Perioperative Standards and Recommended Practices. (2014), Recommended practices:
• Prevention of unplanned hypothermia.
• Transfer of patient care information.
• Prevention of deep vein thrombosis.

Key Words

Behavioral response, beliefs, confidentiality, culture, deep vein thrombosis (DVT), hypothermia, intraoperative, knowledge deficit, patient coping mechanisms, patient education, patient privacy, patient transfer, physiologic response, sequential compression device (SCD), spirituality, stress, time-out, venous stasis

---

Case Study Activity

What intraoperative nursing interventions can be implemented to decrease the risk for the development of a DVT for Mr. J. postoperatively?

Activity — Critical Thinking

Your patient, scheduled for a total hip arthroplasty, has stated that her religious beliefs prevent her from accepting a blood transfusion. What are your choices in fluid management that will respect her wishes?

Case Study Activity

1. Complete the script for Mr. J.'s time-out.

Good morning, this is _____, the circulator for (patient's name).

The consent and H&P state that the scheduled procedure is _____.

The (side/site) has been marked.

X-rays are in the room and confirm (side and site).

Implants for a (site and side) are sterile and available in the room.

Special equipment available includes:_____ and _____.

We can proceed when there is verbal agreement from the team. Are there any questions or concerns?

Verbal agreement ____Yes

Circulator's signature:_____

Continued on next page.

Case Study Activity *(continued)*

2. Mr. J. wonders "what all the fuss is about" concerning keeping him warm. He states, "In 5 minutes, I'll be asleep, and won't even know if I'm cold or not." What do you tell him?

3. From your preoperative assessment, you learn that Mr. J.'s maternal grandfather died during surgery to remove his thyroid. Mr. J. states, "You know, I've had a lot of surgery, but I still wonder if the same thing couldn't happen to me." What nursing interventions can you employ to decrease his anxiety?

4. Physiologic responses to the stress of the surgical procedure and Mr. J.'s health assessment can trigger some unique situations for the management of his care. In reviewing his preoperative assessment, what physiologic responses might you as his intraoperative nurse encounter?

"Go To" Activity — Check It Out!

Go to Question #18, Age-specific care; Question #20, Pediatrics; and Question #42, Alternatives to blood transfusion, under the Perioperative question of the week tab in the Toolbox at http://www.cc-institute.org/toolbox for additional critical-thinking activities.

"Go To" Activity — Skill Building

Review your facility's policies and procedures on prevention of deep vein thrombosis and hypothermia and compare them to AORN's standards and recommended practices.

Identify the resources in your facility that can be used to address your patient's spiritual needs.

Additional Readings/Resources

AORN Human Factors in Health Care Tool Kit. AORN,Inc. Retrieved Feb. 27, 2014, from https://www.aorn.org/Clinical_Practice/ToolKits/Tool_Kits.aspx
Note: Must be an AORN member to access.

Bailey, L. (2010). Strategies for decreasing patient anxiety in the perioperative setting. *AORN Journal*, *92*(4), 445-460.

Griffin, A. (2013). The lived spiritual experiences of patients transitioning through major outpatient surgery. *AORN Journal, 97*(2), 243-252.

Huang, L, Kim, R., & Berry, W. (2013). Creating a culture of safety by using checklists. *AORN Journal, 97*(3), 365-368.

The Joint Commission. VTE prophylaxis options for surgery. Retrieved Jan. 20, 2014, from https://manual.jointcommission.org/pub/Manual/MIF0061/SCIPVTE2_Algorithm.pdf

The Joint Commission. Universal Protocol for Preventing Wrong Site, Wrong Procedure, Wrong Person Surgery. Retrieved Feb. 26, 2014, from http://www.jointcommission.org/assets/1/18/UP_Poster1.pdf

Larkin, B.G., Mitchell, K.M., & Petrie, K. (2012). Translating evidence to practice for mechanical venous thromboembolism prophylaxis. *AORN Journal, 96*(5), 513-527.

Lynch, S., Dixon, J., & Leary, D. (2010). Reducing the risk of unplanned perioperative hypothermia. *AORN Journal, 92*(5), 553-565.

McDowell, D.S., & McComb, S.A. (2014). Safety checklist briefings: A systematic review of the literature. *AORN Journal, 99*(1), 125-137.e13.

Norton, E.K., & Rangel, S.J. (2010). Implementing a pediatric surgical safety checklist in the OR and beyond. *AORN Journal*, *92*(1), 61-71.

Shapiro, F.E., Punwani, N., & Urman, R.D. (2013). Checklist implementation for office-based surgery: A team effort. *AORN Journal, 98*(3), 305-309.

Wu, X. (2013). The safe and efficient use of forced-air warming systems. *AORN Journal, 97*(3), 302-308.

Module 2: Support Safe Practices Regarding Anesthesia Provider, Surgeon, and Nurse Administered Medications

Although the number of drugs actually administered by the perioperative nurse may be quite small, the nurse is still responsible for their safe delivery to the sterile field. The responsibility for choosing the right drug in the right dose for the right patient, given via the right route, at the right time, for the right reason, and with the right documentation, is shared by all members of the surgical team. The perioperative nurse's role and responsibility related to anesthetic management of the intraoperative patient varies in scope, depending upon the presence of an anesthesia care provider, the health status of the patient, and the anesthetic technique employed. As nursing scope of practice expands to administering and monitoring drugs traditionally given by an anesthesia care provider, the perioperative nurse acquires additional skills in assessing and managing the patient undergoing moderate sedation.

Competency Outcomes

To successfully complete the activities in this module, you will need to be able to:

1. Differentiate nursing actions utilized in assisting the anesthesia care provider with regional and general anesthesia.
2. Identify key points in providing safe care for the anesthetized patient.
3. Examine the role of the nurse in monitoring a patient undergoing moderate sedation.
4. Review pharmacology of drugs administered during the intraoperative phase.

Recommended Readings

Alexander's Care of the Patient in Surgery. (2015, 15th ed.), Chapter 2: Patient safety and risk management; Chapter 5: Anesthesia.

Berry and Kohn's Operating Room Technique. (2013, 12th ed.), Chapter 2: Foundations of perioperative patient care standards; Chapter 23: Surgical pharmacology; Chapter 24: Anesthesia: Techniques and agents; Chapter 25: Coordinated roles of the scrub person and the circulating nurse.

Perioperative Standards and Recommended Practices. (2014), Recommended practices:
• Managing the patient receiving moderate sedation/analgesia.
• Medication safety.
• Managing the patient receiving local anesthesia.

Key Words

Action, analgesia, anesthetic, cricoid pressure, delivery, documentation, drugs, labeling, malignant hyperthermia medication, medication reconciliation, moderate sedation, patient safety, pharmacology, physical status classification, physiologic response, seven rights, solutions

Activity — Matching

1. Draw a line between the physical status classification and the corresponding patient.

P1	19 y/o male, motor vehicular accident with brain death, DNR with organ donor card
P2	64-year-old female, history of hypertension (typically runs 150/90 to 165/100 mmHg with medication), BMI 45
P3	72-year-old male, diabetes mellitus type II, COPD, end stage renal disease, oxygen 5L/min nasal cannula
P4	45 y/o female with spontaneous ruptured congenital cerebral aneurysm
P5	22 y/o female, healthy, only medication oral birth control
P6	48-year-old male, diabetes mellitus type II, takes Glyburide. Hemoglobin A1c is 6.9

2. Circle the patients who are appropriate for nurse-monitored moderate sedation.

Activity — Critical Thinking

1. You are caring for an 18-month-old patient undergoing bilateral myringotomy with insertion of ear tubes. The surgeon asks you to give an acetaminophen (Tylenol) suppository. The child weighs 26 pounds. The dose is 10 mg/kg, and the drug is supplied in 80, 120, and 325 mg suppositories.

    A. What is the correct route and dosage for this drug for this patient?

    B. What else will you need to do to correctly administer this drug?

2. You work in a cardiac cath lab and frequently monitor patients undergoing moderate sedation/anesthesia. What monitoring equipment should be provided for safe patient care?

Activity — Do You Know?

You are monitoring a patient undergoing a central venous catheter insertion under moderate sedation. The surgeon asks you to give an initial dose of 3 mg of midazolam (Versed) IV push. You would (circle the correct response):

A. Question the surgeon. The amount is lower than the normal range for the initial recommended dose.

B. Question the surgeon. The amount is higher than the normal range for the initial recommended dose.

C. Give the dose. It is within the normal range for the initial recommended dose.

Activity — Critical Thinking

You are caring for a 17-year-old boy, "Ryan," who has a history of Duchenne muscular dystrophy. He is scheduled for debridement of a pressure ulcer on his sacrum under general anesthesia. Based on his history, what anesthetic(s) should be avoided?

Activity — Short Answer

You are caring for a patient scheduled for a laparoscopic Nissen fundoplication. When you arrive to interview the patient, you find him sitting up at a 90-degree angle. He states that when he lies flat, he "gets terrible heartburn." What is the risk for this patient in undergoing a general anesthetic? What can you anticipate the anesthesiologist will need?

"Go To" Activity — Check It Out!

Go to Question #2, Medication administration; Question #5, Moderate sedation; Question #19, Pharmacology; Question #32, Propofol; and Question #41, Routine discontinuance of aspirin preoperatively, under the Perioperative question of the week tab in the Toolbox at http://www.cc-institute.org/toolbox for additional critical-thinking activities.

"Go To" Activity — Skill Building

Ask your anesthesia provider to provide an in-service, nursing grand rounds, or brown bag on safe practices for the anesthetized patient.

Review your policy on moderate sedation/analgesia and compare it with AORN's recommended practices.

Consult your state board of nursing related to nursing administration of anesthetic drugs.

Review contents of your difficult airway cart or supply box.

Additional Readings/Resources

Cochico, S.G. (2012). Propofol allergy: Assessing for patient risks. *AORN Journal, 96*(4), 398-408.

Hernandez, J., Goeckner, B., & Wanzer, L. (2011). Perioperative pharmacology: Pharmacotherapeutics, pharmacokinetics, and pharmacodynamics. *AORN Journal, 93*(2), 259-269.

Hicks, R.W., Wanzer, L., & Goeckner, B. (2011). Perioperative pharmacology: A framework for perioperative medication safety. *AORN Journal, 93*(1), 136-145.

Hicks, R., Wanzer, L., & Denholm, B. (2012). Implementing AORN recommended practices for medication safety. *AORN Journal, 96*(6), 605-626.

Hudek, K. (2009). Emergence delirium: A nursing perspective. *AORN Journal, 89*(3), 509-520.

Johnson, J. (2008). The increasing incidence of anesthetic adverse events in late afternoon surgeries. *AORN Journal, 88*(1), 79-87.

Mainer, J.A. (2010). Nonpharmacological interventions for assisting the induction of anesthesia in children. *AORN Journal, 92*(2), 209-210.

Malignant Hyperthermia Association of the United States (MHAUS). (2014). Retrieved Feb. 28, 2014, from http://www.mhaus.org/
Note: Excellent resources, videos, and hotline.

Mayne, I.P., & Bagaoisan, C. (2009). Social support during anesthesia induction in an adult surgical population. *AORN Journal, 89*(2), 307-320.

Treiber, L.A., & Jones, J.H. (2012). Medication errors, routines, and differences between perioperative and non-perioperative nurses. *AORN Journal, 96*(3), 285-294.

Wanzer, L., Goeckner, B., & Hicks, R.W. (2011). Perioperative pharmacology: Antibiotic administration. *AORN Journal, 93*(3), 340-351.

Module 3: Incorporate Principles of Safe Positioning

Every patient is positioned with two goals in mind: optimal exposure for the surgeon, and optimal outcomes for the patient. This crucial step carries with it a host of risks and potential complications, which the perioperative nurse, anesthesia provider, and surgeon must anticipate and intervene to prevent.

Competency Outcomes

To successfully complete the activities in this module, you will need to be able to:

1. Describe complications associated with surgical positioning.
2. Select appropriate positioning devices.
3. Choose the correct position based on procedural and patient needs.

Recommended Readings

Alexander's Care of the Patient in Surgery. (2015, 15th ed.), Chapter 2: Patient safety and risk management; Chapter 6: Positioning the patient for surgery.

Berry and Kohn's Operating Room Technique. (2013, 12th ed.), Chapter 2: Foundations of perioperative patient care standards; Chapter 26: Positioning, prepping, and draping the patient.

Perioperative Standards and Recommended Practices. (2014), Recommended practices: Positioning the patient.

Key Words

Braden score, Fowler, lateral, lithotomy, nerve injury, positioning, pressure points, prone, reverse Trendelenburg, semi-Fowler, skin integrity, supine, Trendelenburg

Activity — X Marks the Spot

Mark with an "X" the pressure points associated with the following patient positions.

Supine

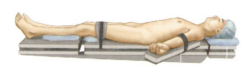

Prone

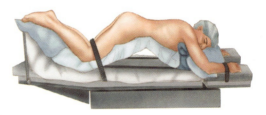

Lithotomy, boot stirrups

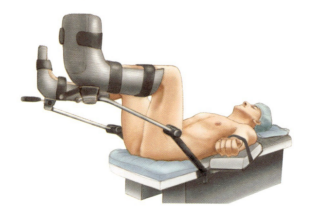

Sitting

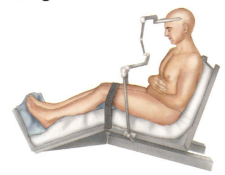

Lateral decubitis

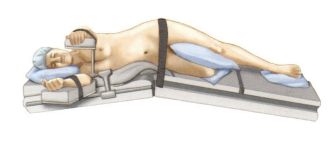

Activity — Circle the Correct Answer

In the left lateral decubitis position, the patient is lying on the _____ side.

RIGHT   LEFT

When positioning a patient for a Cesarean section, the hip roll is placed under the _____ hip to displace the uterus from the inferior vena cava.

RIGHT   LEFT

Activity — Matching

Match the position with the associated nerve injury.
Answers may be used more than once.

Supine _____   A. brachial plexus

Lithotomy _____   B. peroneal

Lateral _____   C. saphenous

Prone _____   D. sciatic

Semi-Fowler _____   E. ulnar

Fowler _____   F. radial

Activity — Do You Know?

The preferred placement for the patient's arms in the prone position is _____.
(circle one)

ON ARMBOARDS   AT THE PATIENT'S SIDES

"Go To" Activity — Skill Building

Locate and review your manufacturers' manuals on the use of positioning devices.

Access your facility's OR bed training manual/video or ask your industry representative to provide this information.

Additional Readings/Resources

"Go To" Activity — Check It Out!

Go to Question #40, Lithotomy positioning, under the Perioperative question of the week tab in the Toolbox at http://www.cc-institute.org/toolbox for an additional critical-thinking activity.

Bennicoff, G. (2010). Perioperative care of the morbidly obese patient in the lithotomy position. *AORN Journal, 92*(3), 297-312.

Bouyer-Ferullo, S. (2013). Preventing peripheral nerve injuries. *AORN Journal, 97*(1), 111-121.

Denholm, B. (2009). Tucking patients' arms and general positioning. *AORN Journal, 89*(4), 755-757.

Munro, C.A. (2010). The development of a pressure ulcer risk-assessment scale for perioperative patients. *AORN Journal, 92*(3), 272-287.

Sutton, S., Link, T., & Makic, M.B.F. (2013). A quality improvement project for safe and effective patient positioning during robotic-assisted surgery. *AORN Journal, 97*(4), 448-456.

Walton-Geer, P.S. (2009). Prevention of pressure ulcers in the surgical patient. *AORN Journal, 89*(3), 538-552.

Module 4: Prepare the Surgical Site

By definition, the surgical incision breaches one of the body's main protective barriers — the skin. Understanding and applying current best practices in patient skin preparation can decrease the risk of surgical site infections.

Competency Outcomes

To successfully complete the activities in this module, you will need to be able to:

1. Classify stages of wound healing.
2. Apply the appropriate skin preparation antiseptic based on skin integrity, number and kinds of contaminants, patient's individual needs (e.g., allergies), and area to be prepped.
3. Choose methods of hair removal based on current best practice.
4. Incorporate components of the Surgical Care Improvement Project (SCIP).

Recommended Readings

Alexander's Care of the Patient in Surgery. (2015, 15th ed.), Chapter 4: Infection prevention and control in the perioperative setting.

Berry and Kohn's Operating Room Technique. (2013, 12th ed.), Chapter 26: Positioning, prepping, and draping the patient.

Perioperative Standards and Recommended Practices. (2014), Recommended practices: Preoperative patient skin antisepsis.

Key Words

Antiseptic, cleansing, prep, skin antisepsis, Surgical Care Improvement Project (SCIP), surgical site, wound healing

Activity — Critical Thinking

You are caring for a patient who is scheduled for reanastomosis of a colostomy. How is the typical skin prep adjusted for this patient?

Activity — Critical Thinking

The surgeon requests that hair be removed from the immediate incisional area for an extremely hirsute male scheduled for an inguinal herniorraphy. What is the best method for accomplishing this?

Case Study Activity

How will Mr. J.'s allergy to shellfish affect the choice of skin antisepsis?

"Go To" Activity — Check It Out!

Go to Question #3, Prepping agents for mucous membranes, and Question #35, Shellfish and prep agents, under the Perioperative question of the week tab in the Toolbox at http://www.cc-institute.org/toolbox for additional critical-thinking activities.

Activity — Color Me

For each illustration below and on the following pages, mark the incision (if applicable) and shade the area to be prepped.

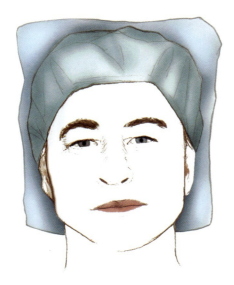

Cataract extraction, right eye

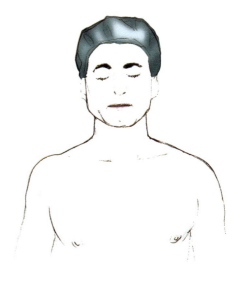

Right carotid endarterectomy

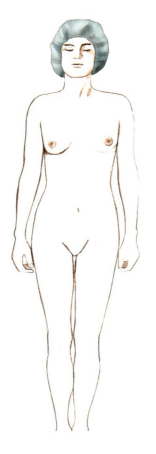

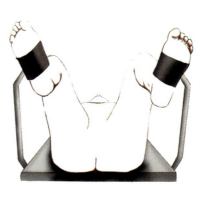

Abdominal/perineal resection

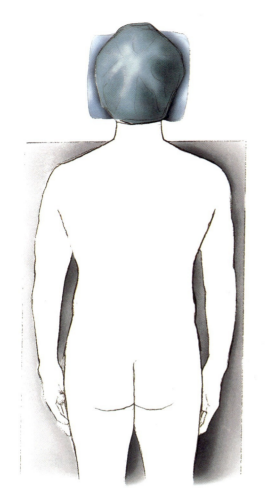

Lumbar discectomy, L4-L5

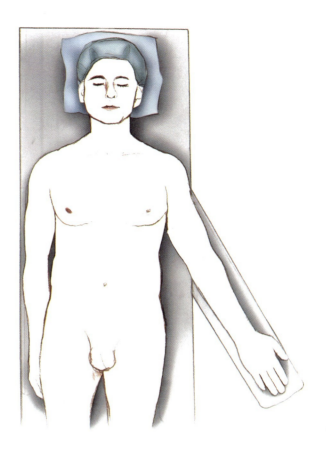

Laparoscopic cholecystectomy

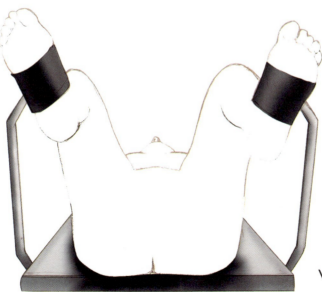

Vaginal hysterectomy

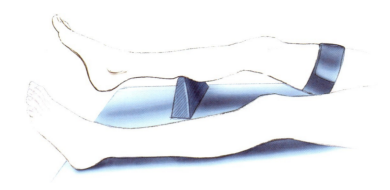

Right bunionectomy

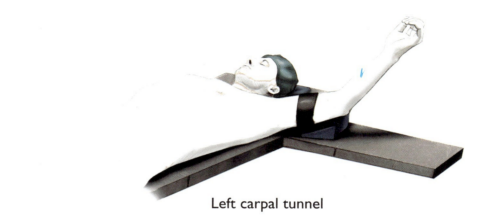

Left carpal tunnel

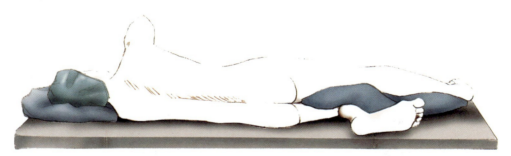

Right nephrectomy

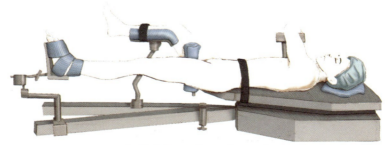

Left hip arthroplasty

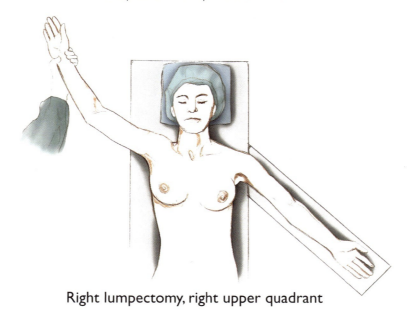

Right lumpectomy, right upper quadrant

For the illustrations above and on the previous three pages, circle the pictures in which chlorhexidine gluconate may be used as the skin prep agent.

"Go To" Activity — Skill Building

Compare your facility's policy and procedure related to patient skin preparation with AORN's recommended practices on patient skin antisepsis.

Additional Readings/Resources

Barnes, S. (2012). In focus: Optimizing and moving beyond SCIP. *AORN Journal, 95*(1), C5-C6.

Burlingame, B. (2011). Clinical issues: Abdominal-perineal surgical preps; Perineal preps and urinary catheter insertion. *AORN Journal, 94*(1), 97-100.

Edmiston, C. E., Okoli, O., Graham, M.B., Sinski, S., et al. (2010). Evidence for using chlorhexidine gluconate preoperative cleansing to reduce the risk of surgical site infection. *AORN Journal, 92*(5), 509-518.

Graling, P.R., & Vasaly, F.W. (2013). Effectiveness of 2% CHG cloth bathing for reducing surgical site infections. *AORN Journal, 97*(5), 547-551.

Hanlan, K.A., McCutcheon, S.P., McCutcheon, J.G., et al. (2013). Quality improvement: Single-field sterile scrub, prep, and dwell for laparoscopic hysterectomy. *AORN Journal, 97*(5), 539-546.

Institute for Healthcare Improvement (IHI). (2013). Surgical site infection. Retrieved Feb. 4, 2014, from http://www.ihi.org/explore/SSI/Pages/default.aspx.

Waters, T., Spera, P., Petersen, C., et al. (2011). AORN Ergonomic Tool 3: Lifting and holding the patient's legs, arms, and head while prepping. *AORN Journal, 93*(5), 589-592.

Zinn, J., Jenkins, J.B., Harrelson, B., et al. (2013). Differences in intraoperative prep solutions: A retrospective chart review. *AORN Journal, 97*(5), 552-558.

Zinn, J., Jenkins, J.B., Swofford, V., Harrelson, B., et al. (2010). Intraoperative patient skin prep agents: Is there a difference? *AORN Journal*, *92*(6), 662-674.

Module 5: Apply Principles of Asepsis

Observing the basic rules of asepsis is the most important action the perioperative nurse can perform in helping to prevent surgical site infections. In addition to being responsible for his/her own actions, the nurse's strong sense of surgical conscience implies holding all members of the surgical care team to those same high standards.

Competency Outcomes

To successfully complete the activities in this module, you will need to be able to:

1. Apply principles of asepsis to perioperative nursing actions.
2. Identify actions to correct breaks in technique.
3. Classify wounds according to Centers for Disease Control and Prevention definitions.

Recommended Readings

Alexander's Care of the Patient in Surgery. (2015, 15th ed.), Chapter 2: Patient safety and risk management; Chapter 4: Infection prevention and control in the perioperative setting.

Berry and Kohn's Operating Room Technique. (2013, 12th ed.), Chapter 2: Foundations of perioperative patient care standards; Chapter 15: Principles of asepsis and sterile techniques; Chapter 16: Appropriate attire, surgical hand cleansing, gowning, and gloving; Chapter 20: Wound healing and hemostasis, p. 577.

Perioperative Standards and Recommended Practices. (2014), Recommended practices:
- Surgical attire.
- Hand hygiene.
- Sterile technique.
- Traffic patterns.
- Product selection.
- Prevention of transmissible infections.

Key Words

Asepsis, gloving, gowning, hand hygiene, sterile field, sterile technique, surgical attire, surgical consciousness, traffic patterns

Activity — Matching

Match the area with the required appropriate attire. Answers may be used more than once.

Cafeteria _____

Sterile supply room _____

OR with opened supplies _____

A. mask
B. surgical scrubs
C. hair covering
D. coverall/jumpsuit
E. street clothes

Activity — Fill In the Blank

For the following procedures, write in the corresponding wound classification:

Total knee replacement: _____

Incision and drainage of abscess, status postop posterior spinal fusion: _____

Appendectomy, unruptured: _____

Open reduction internal fixation open fracture right radius/ulna:_____

Gunshot wound to abdomen: _____

Bowel resection, no spillage: _____

Rhytidectomy: _____

Bowel resection, spillage: _____

Myringotomy: _____

Activity — Critical Thinking

Circle the most effective method for disinfecting hands after caring for a patient with *Clostridium difficile*.

Activity — Short Answer

1. While setting up your room, you drop an unopened box of 4X4 radiopaque sponges on the floor. What is the correct action?

2. You are scrubbed for a laparoscopic cholecystectomy. The surgeon asks you to move to the other side of the table to hold the camera while initiating an additional port site. What is the appropriate way to pass the other scrubbed members of the team?

3. After opening up and counting your sterile field for a laparoscopic-assisted vaginal hysterectomy (LAVH), the charge nurse informs you that the surgeon has an emergency in labor and delivery. Your scrub technician asks if the back table can be covered. What is the correct response?

"Go To" Activity — Check It Out!

Go to Question #15, Surgical attire, and Question #16, Infection control, under the Perioperative question of the week tab in the Study Guide Toolbox at http://www.cc-institute.org/toolbox for critical-thinking questions.

Additional Readings/Resources

Blanchard, J. (2009). Reuse of multidose vials. *AORN Journal, 89*(6), 1128-1129.

Centers for Disease Control and Prevention (CDC). (2014, Jan.). Surgical Site Infection (SSI) Event: Wound classes, p. 9-10. Retrieved Feb. 28, 2014, from http://www.cdc.gov/nhsn/pdfs/pscmanual/9pscssicurrent.pdf

Hopper, W.R., & Moss, R. (2010). Common breaks in sterile technique: Clinical perspectives and perioperative implications. *AORN Journal, 91*(3), 350-367.

Kennedy, L., (2013). Implementing AORN recommended practices for sterile technique. *AORN Journal, 98*(1), 15-23.

Korniewicz, D. & El-Masri, M. (2012). Exploring the benefits of double gloving during surgery. *AORN Journal, 95*(3), 328-336.

Spratt, D., Dutton, R.P., Dellinger, E.P., et al. (2012). The role of the health care professions in preventing surgical site infection. *AORN Journal, 95*(4), 430-440.

Zinn, J. (2012). Surgical wound classification: Communication is needed for accuracy. *AORN Journal, 95*(2), 274-278.

Module 6: Provide Perioperative Nursing Care During Operative and Invasive Procedures

The CNOR exam contains questions related to many different procedures and patient types, some of which may not be familiar to you; therefore, it is highly recommended that you take advantage of opportunities to care for as many different types of patients and procedures as possible in your work setting. Providing examples of every specialty is beyond the scope of this book. By completing the activities, however, you have been provided with the tools to develop your own plan of care for any patient.

Competency Outcomes

To successfully complete the activities in this module, you will need to be able to:

1. Relate pertinent anatomy and physiology to the proposed procedure.
2. Organize a plan of care to accommodate surgical and patient needs.
3. Anticipate and prevent complications inherent to surgery.

Recommended Readings

Alexander's Care of the Patient in Surgery. (2015, 15th ed.), Chapter 4: Infection prevention and control in the perioperative setting; Chapter 7: Sutures, needles, and instruments; Chapter 8: Surgical modalities; Chapter 9: Wound healing, dressings, and drains; Unit II: Surgical interventions; Unit III: Special considerations.

Berry and Kohn's Operating Room Technique. (2013, 12th ed.), Chapter 19: Surgical instrumentation; Chapter 25: Coordinated roles of the scrub person and the circulating nurse; Chapter 28: Surgical incisions, implants, and wound closure; Chapter 29: Wound healing and hemostasis; Chapter 31: Potential perioperative complications; Section 12: Surgical specialties.

Perioperative Standards and Recommended Practices. (2014), Recommended practices:
- Minimally invasive surgery.
- Surgical tissue banking.

Key Words

Anatomy, hemostasis, implant, invasive procedure, minimally invasive, operation, physiology, specialty, surgery, wound healing

"Go To" Case Study Activity

From your previously developed concept map and the patient assessment, develop a plan of care for the intraoperative component of Mr. J.'s perioperative experience.

1. Identify the intraoperative nursing interventions that will need to be implemented for Mr. J.'s surgical procedure. Some of these are typical for every surgery (e.g., infection prevention, principles of aseptic technique, skin antisepsis), while others will be specific for Mr. J.

2. Arrange the intraoperative activities from your list under their corresponding "major problems" boxes you developed in Chapters 1 and 2.

3. At what pressure should the tourniquet be set?

4. Where should the electrosurgical dispersive electrode pad be placed?

Activity — Short Answer

A 17-year-old patient returns to your facility seven months postoperatively for removal of an infected Harrington rod implant. The wound cultures *Staphylococcus aureus*. Is this considered a surgical site infection? Why or why not?

Activity — Name That Incision

Name the abdominal incisions in the diagram on the right.

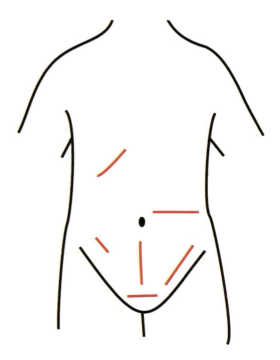

Activity — Matching

Match the incision types listed above to their corresponding surgical procedure. Use each answer only once.

Lower midline _____   A. abdominal hysterectomy

Oblique _____   B. appendectomy

Pfannenstiel _____   C. radical retropubic prostatectomy

Subcostal _____   D. open inguinal herniorraphy

McBurney _____   E. hepatic resection

Transverse _____   F. choledochojejunostomy

Activity — Short Answer

Your patient is scheduled for an ulnar nerve release, left elbow; he states that he has an implantable cardiodefibrillator. What is the safest electrosurgical method to use, and why?

Additional Readings/Resources

Note: Every *AORN Journal* typically includes at least one article on a surgical specialty.

Doerflinger, D.M.C. (2009). Older adult surgical patients: Presentation and challenges. *AORN Journal, 90*(2), 223-244.

Hicks, R.W., and Denholm, B. (2013). Implementing AORN recommended practices for care of patients undergoing pneumatic tourniquet-assisted procedures. *AORN Journal, 98*(4), 153-166.

Roesler, R., Halowell, C.C., Elias, G., & Peters, J. (2010). Chasing zero: Our journey to preventing surgical site infections. *AORN Journal, 91*(2), 224-231.

Ulmer, B. (2010). Best practices for minimally invasive procedures. *AORN Journal, 91*(5), 558-575.

Walters, L., & Eley, S. (2011). Robotic-assisted surgery and the need for standardized pathways and clinical guidelines. *AORN Journal, 93*(4), 455-463.

Module 7: Identify and Control Environmental Factors

Managing intraoperative environmental factors (e.g., temperature, humidity, traffic flow, noise) contributes to optimal patient outcomes. The push for shorter turnover times should not compromise room cleaning, which is frequently performed by unlicensed assistive personnel with limited knowledge of transmission of infectious agents or antiseptic principles. It is ultimately the perioperative nurse's responsibility to ensure that the intraoperative environment is safe and meets facility and regulatory standards for providing safe patient care.

Competency Outcomes

To successfully complete the activities in this module, you will need to be able to:

1. Select normal values for air exchanges, humidity, and temperature.
2. Apply principles of antisepsis to maintenance of a clean environment.

Recommended Readings

Alexander's Care of the Patient in Surgery. (2015, 15th ed.), Chapter 4: Infection prevention and control in the perioperative setting.

AORN. (2009). Position statement on noise in the perioperative practice setting. Retrieved Feb. 4, 2014, from http://www.aorn.org/Clinical_Practice/Position_Statements/Position_Statements. aspx.

Berry and Kohn's Operating Room Technique. (2013, 12th ed.), Chapter 10: Physical facilities; Chapter 11: Ambulatory surgery centers and alternative surgery locations; Chapter 12: Care of the intraoperative environment; Chapter 13: Potential sources of injury to the caregiver and the patient.

Perioperative Standards and Recommended Practices. (2014), Recommended practices:
- Environmental cleaning in the perioperative setting.
- Safe environment of care.

Key Words

Air exchanges, antiseptic, environmental cleaning, humidity, infectious waste, noise, room turnover, spills, temperature, terminal cleaning, traffic patterns, turnover

Activity — Fill In the Blank

For each of the following environmental controls, list the acceptable parameters:

Air exchanges:

OR:_____ Cardiac cath lab:_____ Sterile storage area: _____

Decontamination area: _____

Humidity:

OR:_____ Cardiac cath lab:_____ Decontamination area: _____

Temperature:

OR:_____ Cardiac cath lab:_____ Decontamination area: _____

Air pressure in the OR should be _____ than the surrounding corridors.
(greater/lower)

Activity — Short Answer

For each source of noise, list a nursing intervention to reduce its risk of disrupting the environment and impacting patient safety:

Beeper/pager/cell phone:

Monitor alarms:

Electronic music devices (radios, CD players):

Overhead pages and announcements:

Telephones:

Staff communication:

Case Study Activity

As the anesthesia care provider hands you a tube of blood for a blood chemistry analysis for Mr. J., it slips out of your hand and drops to the floor, breaking the tube. What is the best way to clean up the spill?

"Go To" Activity — Skill Building

Compare how your facility monitors and documents OR air exchange rates, temperature, and humidity with AORN standards and recommended practices.

"Go To" Activity — Check It Out!

Go to Question #11, Infection Control, under the Perioperative question of the week tab in the Toolbox at http://www.cc-institute.org/toolbox for a critical-thinking question related to cleaning a room after a patient infected with MRSA.

Activity — Critical Thinking

How does end of procedure (turnover) cleaning between cases differ from that done at the end of the day (terminal cleaning)?

Additional Readings/Resources

Blanchard, J. (2009). Terminal cleaning. *AORN Journal, 89*(2), 409-411.

Chen, L., Brueck, S.E., & Niemeier, M.T. (2012). Evaluation of potential noise exposure in hospital operating rooms. *AORN Journal, 96*(4), 412-418.

Clark, G.J. (2013). Strategies for preventing distractions and interruptions in the OR. *AORN Journal, 97*(6), 702-707.

Jefferson, J., Whelan, R., Dick, B., & Carling, P. (2011). A novel technique for identifying opportunities to improve environmental hygiene in the operating room. *AORN Journal, 93*(3), 358-364.

Kohut, K. (2010). Infection prevention in the interventional settings. Retrieved March 1, 2014, from http://www.apicchicago.org/pdf/2010/Interventional_IP_KK_%2010-8-10.pdf

VandeLeest, L., Kawczynski, R., Lipp, F.E., et al. (2012). Identifying potential areas of infectivity on high-touch locations in the OR. *AORN Journal, 96*(5), 507-512.

Module 8: Monitor and Intervene to Reduce the Risk of Complications and Adverse Outcomes

A variety of equipment unique to the OR contributes to maintaining the high level of technologically sophisticated care enjoyed by today's surgical patient. This same equipment also holds inherent risks that must be safely managed to avoid injury to both patients and staff.

Competency Outcomes

To successfully complete the activities in this module, you will need to be able to:

1. Identify common hazards associated with the intraoperative environment.
2. Recognize the importance of following manufacturers' recommendations for safely operating their equipment.

Recommended Readings

Alexander's Care of the Patient in Surgery. (2015, 15th ed.), Chapter 2: Patient safety and risk management; Chapter 3: Workplace issues and staff safety.

AORN. (2011). Position statement: Creating a practice environment of safety. Retrieved March 1, 2014, from http://www.aorn.org/Clinical_Practice/Position_Statements/Position_Statements.aspx

Berry and Kohn's Operating Room Technique. (2013, 12th ed.), Chapter 2: Foundations of perioperative patient care standards; Chapter 13: Potential sources of injury to the caregiver and patient; Chapter 20: Specialized surgical equipment; Chapter 22: Diagnostic procedures and oncologic considerations; Chapter 27: Physiologic maintenance and monitoring of the perioperative patient; Chapter 31: Potential perioperative complications.

Perioperative Standards and Recommended Practices. (2014), Recommended practices:
- Electrosurgery.
- Laser safety in perioperative practice settings.
- Pneumatic tourniquet.
- Reducing radiological exposure.
- Sharps injury prevention.

Key Words

Adverse event, body mechanics, chemicals, electrosurgery, equipment testing, ergonomics, fire, laser, National Patient Safety Goals, patient safety, radiation, sharps injury, smoke evacuation

Activity — Fill in the Blank

The three principles related to radiation protection are _____,

_____, and _____.

Activity — Critical Thinking

1. You are the circulating nurse for an 11-year-old boy undergoing an open reduction internal fixation for a right malleolar fracture from a skate-board accident. You notice that the tourniquet time is approaching 60 minutes. What action, if any, needs to be taken?

2. Your patient is scheduled for a laser tonsillectomy. What safety mechanisms should be in place to care for your patient?

Activity — Critical Thinking

What interventions can be implemented to safely transfer a patient scheduled for a laparascopic Roux-en-Y gastric bypass procedure?

Case Study Activity

1. Dr. S. repeatedly asks for the coagulation power on the electrosurgical unit to be increased. What steps should be taken in trouble-shooting a possible problem?

2. Upon completion of the surgery, a slightly reddened area is noted under the site for Mr. J.'s electrosurgical dispersive electrode pad. What steps need to be taken in treating and reporting this incident?

"Go To" Activity — Skill Building

Talk with your facility quality department or laser safety officer about the most current safety standards regarding use of lasers in your facility.

Compare your policy on laser use with AORN's recommended practices.

Check with your industry representative who supplies your electrosurgical equipment and supplies for educational materials on dispersive electrode safety and adverse effects of surgical smoke plume exposure.

Ask the radiation safety officer at your facility to provide a staff in-service to discuss patient and staff radiation safety issues, including what staff can do to promote safe practices when exposed to radiation in the OR. Ask for information on the proper way to wear monitoring badges based on facility and state standards.

Ask your risk mitigation officer to review your facility's policy on occurrence reporting.

Additional Readings/Resources

Blanchard, J. (2009). Protecting personnel who work with radiation. *AORN Journal*, *89*(6), 1127-1128.

Fred, C., Ford, S., Wagner, D., et al. (2012). Intraoperatively acquired pressure ulcers and perioperative normothermia: A look at relationships. *AORN Journal, 96*(3), 251-260.

Graham, D., Faggionato, E., & Timberlake, A. (2011). Preventing perioperative complications in the patient with a high body mass index. *AORN Journal, 94*(4), 334-347.

Smith, F.D. (2010). Management of exposure to waste anesthetic gases. *AORN Journal, 91*(4), 482-494.

Vose, J.G,. & Adara-Berkowitz, J. (2009). Reducing scalpel injuries in the operating room. *AORN Journal, 90*(6), 867-872.

Watson, D. (2010). Radiation safety. *AORN Journal, 92*(2), 233-235.

Watson, D. (2010). Surgical smoke evacuation during laparoscopic surgery. *AORN Journal, 92*(3), 347-350.

Module 9: Prepare and Label Specimens

Although tissue, body fluids, and bone typically come to mind when specimens are discussed, a specimen is anything removed from a patient's body. In addition to assisting in providing a diagnosis, the results of specimen analysis may influence the course of treatment, the need for additional procedures, and forensic evidence.

Competency Outcomes

To successfully complete the activities in this module, you will need to be able to:

1. Prepare a specimen for transport to the laboratory.
2. Describe items to include in identification of a specimen.

Recommended Readings

Alexander's Care of the Patient in Surgery. (2015, 15th ed.), Chapter 2: Patient safety and risk management.

Berry and Kohn's Operating Room Technique. (2013, 12th ed.), Chapter 2: Foundations of perioperative patient care standards, p. 26; Chapter 22: Diagnostics, specimens, and oncologic considerations; Chapter 25: Coordinated roles of the scrub person and the circulating nurse.

Perioperative Standards and Recommended Practices. (2014), Recommended practices: Care and handling of specimens in the perioperative environment.

Key Words

Culture, documentation, explanted medical device, handling, implanted medical device, specimen, tissue tracking

Activity — Short Answer

Identification of the specimen should be confirmed verbally between the circulating nurse and the surgeon using a "read back" communication similar to that used with verbal orders. What information needs to be communicated between the surgeon and circulating nurse?

Activity — True or False

1. As long as an instrument is used to transfer the specimen from the sterile field to the specimen jar, the circulator is not required to wear gloves or eye protection.

TRUE   FALSE

2. The specimen label should be placed on the lid of the container.

TRUE   FALSE

"Go To" Activity — Skill Building

Take a field trip to your laboratory. Ask to observe how different tissues are processed.

Review your facility's policy on processing explanted medical devices; how does it differ from AORN recommended practices?

"Go To" Activity — Check It Out!

Go to Question #14, Specimen handling, and Question #31, Forensics, under the Perioperative question of the week tab in the Toolbox at http://www.cc-institute.org/toolbox for critical-thinking activities.

Module 10: Perform Counts

Retained surgical items (RSIs) cause unnecessary pain and suffering to the patient and additional expense to the health care facility. RSIs are considered a sentinel or "never event" and are required to be reported to The Joint Commission. A primary goal of performing counts is to avoid RSIs by providing consistent, standardized, and achievable methods for accounting for suture, instruments, and sharps. Sponges, sharps and miscellaneous items should be counted for every procedure; instruments should be counted whenever there is a possibility of losing an item (AORN, 2014).

Competency Outcomes

To successfully complete the activities in this module, you will need to be able to:

1. Identify appropriate items to be counted at the correct time.
2. Describe the correct action to take for an incorrect count.

Recommended Readings

Alexander's Care of the Patient in Surgery. (2015, 15th ed.), Chapter 2: Patient safety and risk management; Chapter 7: Sutures, needles, and instruments.

Berry and Kohn's Operating Room Technique. (2013, 12th ed.), Chapter 2: Foundations of perioperative patient care standards; Chapter 25: Coordinated roles of the scrub person and the circulating nurse.

Perioperative Standards and Recommended Practices. (2014), Recommended practices: Prevention of retained surgical items.

Key Words

Closing, complication, count, instruments, miscellaneous items, needles, retained item, sharps, sponges

Activity — Do You Know?

How many strategies can you list to help prevent a retained surgical item?

Activity — Critical Thinking

You are counting sponges with the scrub person in preparation for an abdominal hysterectomy. The package of 4X4 radiopaque sponges you have opened contains 9 sponges instead of 10. What should you do?

Activity — Scramble

Number the following steps in the correct order for completing a sponge and suture count:

_____ When wound (peritoneum) closure begins

_____ Before the procedure

_____ At skin closure

_____ Before closure of a cavity (e.g., uterus or bladder) within a cavity

List three other circumstances when a count should be performed:

1._____ 2._____ 3._____

Case Study Activity

Mr. J.'s surgery is near completion. As a needle holder and needle were returned to the scrub person, he noted that the needle was bent with the tip of the needle missing. Explain your immediate course of action to prevent a retained surgical item. How would you document these issues and the patient care you provided?

"Go To" Activity — Skill Building

Compare your facility's policy and procedure on preventing retained items to AORN's standards and recommended practices.

Ask your risk mitigation manager to provide an in-service on the tools used to investigate an event related to a retained surgical item, e.g., root cause analysis (RCA), failure mode effects analysis (FMEA), etc.

Ask your radiologist to provide an in-service on the process for requesting radiographs for retained surgical items. Ask him/her to bring films of RSIs.

Additional Readings/Resources

Edel, E.M. (2012). Surgical count practice variability and the potential for retained surgical items. *AORN Journal, 95*(2), 228-238.

Edel, E. M. (2010). Increasing patient safety and surgical team communication by using a count/time out board. *AORN Journal, 92*(4), 420-424.

Mitchell, S. (2009). Placing count sheets in instrument trays. *AORN Journal, 90*(2), 280-281.

Norton, E.K., Martin, C., & Micheli, A.J. (2012). Patients count on it: An initiative to reduce incorrect counts and prevent retained surgical items. *AORN Journal, 95*(1), 109.

Rowlands, A. (2012). Risk factors associated with incorrect surgical counts. *AORN Journal, 96* (3), 272-284.

Rowlands, A., & Steeves, R. (2010). Incorrect sponge counts: A qualitative analysis. *AORN Journal, 92*(4), 410-419.

"Go To" Activity Check It Out!

Go to Question #1, Counts, under the Perioperative question of the week tab in the Toolbox at http://www.cc-institute.org/toolbox for a critical-thinking question.

Module 11: Maintain Accurate Patient Records

Many medical errors are due to incomplete or inaccurately documented patient data. One of the goals behind the current movement to record patient information electronically is to provide a standardized framework for documenting data that makes it more difficult to input information incorrectly or not at all. Regardless of the method used, maintenance of accurate patient information related to the surgical experience requires careful attention to detail and should go beyond "checking the boxes." In addition to providing a history of the patient's intraoperative experience, this information will be used as a reference for other health care providers; for quality improvement projects and billing; for reordering of implants, prostheses, and supplies; as a measure of meeting benchmarks for regulatory surveys; and as evidence in a court of law.

Competency Outcomes

To successfully complete the activities in this module, you will need to be able to:

1. Identify data elements to be included in an intraoperative patient record.
2. Use information found in patient records to improve quality of care.

Recommended Readings

Alexander's Care of the Patient in Surgery. (2015, 15th ed.), Chapter 2: Patient safety and risk management.

Berry and Kohn's Operating Room Technique. (2013, 12th ed.), Chapter 2: Foundations of perioperative patient care standards; Chapter 3: Legal, regulatory, and ethical issues; Chapter 11: Ambulatory surgery centers and alternative surgical locations; Chapter 25: Coordinated roles of the scrub person and the circulating nurse.

Perioperative Standards and Recommended Practices. (2014), Recommended practices: Information management.

Key Words

Confidentiality, documentation, electronic medical record (EMR), patient record

Activity — Critical Thinking

You work in a free-standing ambulatory surgery center that enjoys a thriving plastic surgery practice. Your facility has just received a letter from the FDA recalling a certain brand of breast implant. What information from the patients' records do you need to have in determining which of your patients are affected by this recall?

Additional Reading/ Resources

Beach, M.J., & Sions, J.A. (2011). Surviving OR computerization. *AORN Journal, 93*(2), 226-241.

Brusco, J.M. (2011). Electronic health records: What nurses need to know. AORN Journal 93(3), 371-379.

"Go To" Activity — Skill Building

Compare your facility's patient record with the suggested examples in AORN's recommended practices. How do they differ?

Volunteer to serve on a quality improvement committee or chart audit project.

Chapter Summary

Caring for the patient in the intraoperative phase requires a highly developed combination of knowledge and skills that is unique to this specialty. This chapter reviewed the key aspects of intraoperative nursing activities as they relate to the safety, physical, psychological, and sociocultural issues included in the patient's surgical experience. Commitment to quality patient care by implementing current best practices is highlighted.

Glossary

AORN Perioperative Standards and Recommended Practices — As used in the Job Analysis, this term includes all sections of the *Perioperative Standards and Recommended Practices,* published annually by AORN. The most current edition should be used at all times.

Association for the Advancement of Medical Instrumentation (AAMI) — An organization with the goal of increasing the understanding and beneficial use of medical instrumentation. AAMI is the primary source of consensus and timely information on medical instrumentation and technology and is the primary resource for national and international standards for industry, professional organizations, and government agencies. (www.aami.org)

Association of periOperative Registered Nurses (AORN) — AORN is the professional organization of perioperative registered nurses that supports registered nurses in achieving optimal outcomes for patients undergoing operative and other invasive procedures. (www.aorn.org)

Centers for Disease Control and Prevention (CDC) — The federal government agency dedicated to monitoring disease, mortality, and morbidity of patients in the United States. This agency sets guidelines for dealing with known or suspected diseases. The CDC serves as the national focus for developing and applying disease prevention and control, environmental health, and health promotion and education activities designed to improve the health of the people of the United States. (www.cdc.gov)

Cultural diversity — Backgrounds, beliefs, values, and ethnicities that play a major role in communication and interactions between patients and perioperative nurses. Every patient must be evaluated for individual cultural considerations in the perioperative setting.

Delegation — The transfer of responsibility for the performance of an activity from one individual to another while retaining accountability for the outcome.

Domain (related to the PNDS) — The four overall divisions of the conceptual framework of the *Perioperative Nursing Data Set.* All interventions and expected outcomes relate to one or more domain(s). The four domains are Safety, Physiologic Responses, Behavioral Responses, and the Health System.

Healthcare Insurance Portability and Accountability Act (HIPAA) — Legislation passed in 1996 that addresses various aspects of the use of patients' medical information, including confidentiality of patient information in the medical record, consent processes for access to patients' health information, and the right to sue the health plan provider.

Hypothermia — A body temperature significantly below normal (i.e., 98.6° F [37° C]).

May be caused by the operating room environment (e.g., room temperature, exposed skin) and can interfere with patient's maintenance of a normal physiologic state.

Informed consent — The patient's right to make his or her own informed decisions based on information regarding treatment options, including the benefits, expected outcomes, and risk and potential complications; right to refuse treatment; and decisions regarding participation in research studies.

Intervention (nursing) — Action taken, based on patient assessment data, with the intention of achieving one or more expected patient outcomes.

Intraoperative phase — Begins when the patient is transferred to the operating room bed and ends when he or she is admitted to the postanesthesia care unit.

Outcome criteria — Statements developed to identify the tasks or conditions to be implemented that will assist the patient in achieving the desired outcomes. Outcome criteria indicate an expected, measurable change in the patient's health status.

Patients' rights — The rights of every patient to seek and receive health care regardless of his or her race, religion, or culture and with respect for the individual's self-image, privacy, and other such considerations, in accordance with the Patients' Bill of Rights.

Perioperative Nursing Data Set (PNDS) — The perioperative nursing vocabulary guidebook that provides nursing diagnoses, nursing interventions, and patient outcomes statements specific to the perioperative environment.

Perioperative period — Time commencing with the decision for surgical intervention and ending with a follow-up home or clinical evaluation. This period includes the preoperative, intraoperative, and postoperative phases.

Plan of care (or care plan) — A result of a systematic process of identifying expected patient outcomes and determining how to achieve them. It includes the list of interventions necessary to reach the expected outcome. The plan of care directs all nursing care activities related to each patient.

Primary intention — The desired form of wound healing, in which no tissue loss, strict adherence to aseptic technique, and close approximation of wound edges allow for optimal healing with minimal formation of scar tissue.

Regulatory standards — CDC and Occupational Safety and Health Administration regulations and standards and federal, state, and local laws and regulations that govern practice.

Safe environment — The setting in which the physical and psychological aspects of the environment are controlled for the purpose of presenting the least possible hazard to the patient, staff members, and community.

Sentinel event — An unexpected occurrence involving death or serious physical or psychological injury, or the risk thereof.

Surgical intervention — The patient's experiences during the preoperative, intraoperative, and postoperative phases, including the technical aspects and anatomical approach.

Surgical procedure — The technical aspects and anatomical approach used during surgical intervention.

Teaching and learning theories and techniques — Those aids and methods that facilitate learning (e.g., audiovisual tools, return demonstration, adult learning principles).

Terminal cleaning — Thorough cleaning and disinfection of the perioperative environment at the end of daily use.

Transfer — Moving a patient from one place to another (e.g., to or from a bed or stretcher).

Transport — Moving a patient via a device (e.g., wheelchair, stretcher).

Turnover — Cleaning and preparation of the OR between cases for the next patient's arrival.

Universal Protocol Time-Out — As an integral component of The Joint Commission's Universal Protocol for Preventing Wrong Site, Wrong Procedure, Wrong Person Surgery, time-out surgical site verification must be conducted in the location where the procedure will be done, just before starting the procedure. It must involve the entire operative team, use active communication, be briefly documented, and include, at the least
- Correct patient identity
- Correct side and site
- Agreement on the procedure to be done
- Correct patient position
- Availability of correct implants and any special equipment or requirements
Processes and systems should be in place for reconciling differences in staff responses during the time-out.

Unlicensed assistive personnel — Individuals who are trained to function in an assistive role to the registered nurse in providing patient care activities as delegated by, and under the supervision of, the registered nurse.

World Health Organization (WHO) — The directing and coordinating authority for health within the United Nations system. It is responsible for providing leadership on global health matters, shaping the health research agenda, setting norms and standards, articulating evidence-based policy options, providing technical support to countries, and monitoring and assessing health trends.

WHO Safe Surgery Checklist — A checklist that identifies three phases of an operation, each corresponding to a specific period in the normal flow of work: Before the induction of anesthesia (sign in), before the incision of the skin (time-out), and before the patient leaves the operating room (sign out). In each phase, a checklist coordinator must confirm that the surgical team has completed the listed tasks before it proceeds with the operation.

References

AORN. (2014). *Perioperative Standards and Recommended Practices*. Denver: AORN, Inc.

AORN. (2011). *Perioperative Nursing Data Set* (3rd ed.). Denver: AORN, Inc.

Association for the Advancement of Medical Instrumentation. About AAMI. Retrieved April 2, 2013, from http://www.aami.org/about/index.html

Centers for Disease Control and Prevention (CDC).(2013). Healthcare-associated infections (HAIs). Retrieved March 1, 2014, from http://www.cdc.gov/hai/

Institute for Health Improvement (IHI). (2011). World Health Organization (WHO) surgical safety checklist and getting started kit. Retrieved March 1, 2014, from http://www.ihi.org/resources/Pages/Tools/WHOSurgicalSafetyChecklistGettingStartedKit.aspx *Note*: includes a conference call recording, checklist, starter kit, and implementation manual. Registration is required to access documents, but is free and includes a weekly e-newsletter.

Malignant Hyperthermia Association of the United States (MHAUS). (2014). Retrieved Feb. 28, 2014, from http://www.mhaus.org/ Note: Excellent resources, videos, and hotline.

Odom-Forren, J. & Watson, D. (2005). *Practical Guide to Moderate Sedation/Analgesia* (2nd ed.). St. Louis: Elsevier Mosby.

Phillips, N. (2013). *Berry and Kohn's Operating Room Technique* (12th ed.). St. Louis: Mosby.

Rothrock, J.C. (Ed.). (2015). *Alexander's Care of the Patient in Surgery* (15th ed.). St. Louis: Mosby.

World Health Organization (WHO). (2014). WHO surgical safety checklist and implementation manual. Retrieved March 1, 2014, from http://www.who.int/patientsafety/safesurgery/ss_checklist/en/

Answers to Chapter 3 Activities

Module 1: Introduction of the patient to the operative/procedural area — Pages 84-87

Case Study Activity

What intraoperative nursing interventions can be implemented to decrease the risk for the development of a DVT for Mr. J. postoperatively?

Communicate Mr. J.'s high risk for development of a DVT to other health care team members. Organize intraoperative care to decrease tourniquet and surgical time. Implement components of the DVT protocol as appropriate. Ensure sequential compression device is on and working for non-operative leg.

Source: AORN. (2014). Recommended practices for prevention of deep vein thrombosis. In *Perioperative Standards and Recommended Practices*, pp. 422-425. Denver: AORN, Inc.

Activity — Critical Thinking

Your patient, scheduled for a total hip arthroplasty, has stated that her religious beliefs prevent her from accepting a blood transfusion. What are your choices in fluid management that will respect her wishes?

Consider having available volume expanders (colloids and crystalloids) and an autotransfusion (cell salvage) device. Colloids (Albumin, Dextran, Hespan, etc.) and crystalloids (e.g., normal saline, lactated ringers) will assist with maintaining blood pressure but do not have oxygen carrying capabilities. Efficient use of surgical time and hemostasis will also assist in minimizing blood loss.

Source: Rothrock, J.C. (Ed.). (2015). *Alexander's Care of the Patient in Surgery* (15th ed., pp. 36, 38). St. Louis: Mosby.

Case Study Activity

1. Complete the script for Mr. J.'s time-out.
Good morning, this is *(your name)*, the circulator for *Mr. J.*
The consent and H&P state that the scheduled procedure is *left total knee arthroplasty.*
The *left knee* has been marked.
X-rays are in the room and confirm *left knee.*
Implants for a *left total knee* are sterile and available in the room.
Special equipment available (sample): *Sequential compression device; tourniquet; positioning device for operative leg; warm air blanket.*

We can proceed when there is verbal agreement from the team. Are there any questions or concerns?

Verbal agreement: _X_ Yes   Circulator's signature:_____

Source: Rothrock, J. (2015). *Alexander's Care of the Patient in Surgery* (15th ed., pp. 23, 29). St. Louis: Mosby.

2. Mr. J. wonders "what all the fuss is about" concerning keeping him warm. He states, "In 5 minutes, I'll be asleep, and won't even know if I'm cold or not." What do you tell him?

(Sample response; you may think of others)
Being cold is one of the most common complications of surgery. It increases the risk for getting an infection postoperatively, and may promote abnormal heart rates (ventricular tachycardia). It increases the risk for bleeding (inhibits platelet aggregation). It affects the way your body responds to medications so that it takes longer for you to wake up (alters metabolism, increases length of action of muscle relaxant). Because of your age, you're at risk for being cold anyway.

Source: AORN. (2014). Recommended practices for the prevention of hypothermia. In *Perioperative Standards and Recommended Practices*, pp. 431-432. Denver: AORN, Inc.

3. From your preoperative assessment you learn that Mr. J.'s maternal grandfather died during surgery to remove his thyroid. Mr. J. states, "You know, I've had a lot of surgery, but I still wonder if the same thing couldn't happen to me." What nursing interventions can you employ to decrease his anxiety?

(Sample response; yours may vary)
Concerns about dying during surgery should be taken seriously. This information should be communicated to Mr. J.'s surgeon and anesthesiologist.

If Mr. J. agrees, a hospital chaplain or his own spiritual advisor could be asked to talk with him preoperatively.

Nursing interventions to decrease your patient's anxiety include:

*   *Answer questions and provide information in language that Mr. J. can understand.*
*   *Remain in close proximity to provide reassurance.*
*   *Maintain a quiet environment that is focused on Mr. J.*
*   *Introduce other team members and briefly describe their roles.*
*   *Provide privacy by keeping Mr. J. covered and warm.*
*   *Limit traffic in the room.*
*   *Allow Mr. J. to keep his hearing aids as long as possible to enable him to communicate with his caregivers.*

Source: Phillips, N. (2013). *Berry and Kohn's Operating Room Technique* (12th ed., pp. 17, 102, 103, 375, 380). St. Louis: Mosby.

4. Physiologic responses to the stress of the surgical procedure and Mr. J.'s health assessment can trigger some unique situations for the management of his care. In reviewing his preoperative assessment, what physiologic responses might you as his intraoperative nurse encounter?

1. Mr. J.'s age, use of Prednisone, and positioning/use of tourniquet increase his risk for skin breakdown. Careful attention to skin assessment, positioning, and padding will need to be initiated to prevent a break in skin integrity.

2. Mr. J.'s history of GERD may require additional interventions during intubation to prevent aspiration.

3. Major orthopedic surgery and Mr. J.'s meds increase risk for intraoperative bleeding. Borderline low hemoglobin and hematocrit levels may necessitate blood replacement.

4. Mr. J.'s age and the use of a tourniquet will increase his risk for hypothermia. Monitoring of temperature during surgery and the use of a forced warm-air blanket should be implemented.

5. Mr. J's previous DVT, his history of Crohn disease, and the surgical procedure put him at increased risk for a postoperative DVT. Protocols should be followed for prophylaxis.

Module 2: Support safe practices regarding anesthesia provider, surgeon, and nurse administered medications — Pages 88-91

Activity — Matching

1. Draw a line between the physical status classification and the corresponding patient.

P1 = *22 y/o female, healthy, only medication oral birth control*

P2 = *48-year-old male, diabetes mellitus Type II, takes Glyburide. Hemoglobin A1c is 6.9*

P3 = *64-year-old female, history of hypertension (typically runs 150/90 to 165/100 mmHg with medication), BMI 45*

P4 = *72-year-old male, diabetes mellitus Type II, COPD, end stage renal disease, oxygen 5L/min nasal cannula*

P5 = *45 y/o female with spontaneous ruptured congenital cerebral aneurysm*

P6 = *19 y/o male, motor vehicular accident with brain death, DNR with organ donor card*

2. Circle the patients appropriate for nurse-monitored moderate sedation.

Circle patients P1 and P2 (P3 is not medically stable).

> Source: AORN. (2014). Recommended practices for managing the patient receiving moderate sedation/analgesia. In *Perioperative Standards and Recommended Practices*, p. 472. Denver: AORN, Inc.

Activity — Critical Thinking

1. You are caring for an 18-month-old patient undergoing bilateral myringotomy with insertion of ear tubes. The surgeon asks you to give an acetaminophen (Tylenol) suppository. The child weighs 26 pounds. The dose is 10 mg/kg, and the drug is supplied in 80, 120, and 325 mg suppositories.

A. What is the correct route and dosage for this drug for this patient?

Rectal; 26 pounds = 11.8 kg X 10 mg = 118 mg of drug needed.
Administer the 120 mg suppository.

B. What else will you need to do to correctly administer this drug?

Confirm patient identity and presence of any allergies or contraindications. Confirm weight-based dosing and "read back" the order before administration. Use hand hygiene before and after administration of the suppository. Wear a non-sterile glove, and moisten the end of the suppository to ease insertion. Document order and drug, dose, route, and time given in patient record.

Source: AORN. (2014). Recommended practices for medication safety. In *Perioperative Standards and Recommended Practices*, pp. 284-285, 287, 291-292, 301-302. Denver: AORN, Inc.

2. You work in a cardiac cath lab and frequently monitor patients undergoing moderate sedation/anesthesia. What monitoring equipment should be provided for safe patient care?

The recommended equipment for monitoring a patient undergoing moderate sedation is the same regardless of setting. Blood pressure, EKG, and oxygen saturation monitors should be used for every patient. Respiratory rate, pulse rate and rhythm, blood pressure, oxygen saturation, level of consciousness, and skin condition should be monitored at least every 15 minutes throughout the procedure, and after administration of every medication.

Source: Rothrock, J.C. (Ed.). (2015). *Alexander's Care of the Patient in Surgery* (15th ed., p. 149). St. Louis: Mosby.

Activity — Do You Know?

You are monitoring a patient undergoing a central venous catheter insertion under moderate sedation. The surgeon asks you to give an initial dose of 3 mg of midazolam (Versed) IV push. You would (circle the correct response):

A. Question the surgeon. The amount is lower than the normal range for the initial recommended dose.
B. Question the surgeon. The amount is higher than the normal range for the initial recommended dose.
C. Give the dose. It is within the normal range for the initial recommended dose.

B. The normal range for the initial dose for this drug is 1.5-2 mg. The initial titrated dose should not exceed 2.5 mg.

Source: Odom-Forren, J. & Watson, D. (2005). *Practical Guide to Moderate Sedation/Analgesia* (2nd ed., p. 62). St. Louis: Mosby.

Activity — Critical Thinking

You are caring for a 17-year-old boy, "Ryan," with a history of Duchenne muscular dystrophy. He is scheduled for debridement of a pressure ulcer on his sacrum under general anesthesia. Based on his history, what anesthetic(s) should be avoided?

Succinylcholine should always be avoided in patients with Duchenne muscular dystrophy. In addition, consider avoiding anesthetic triggers for malignant hyperthermia, as they may precipitate an MH-like reaction.

Source: Malignant Hyperthermia Association of the United States (MHAUS). (2014). Health care professionals: How to be prepared. Retrieved Feb. 28, 2014, from http://www.mhaus.org/healthcare-professionals/be-prepared/

Activity — Short Answer

1. You are caring for a patient scheduled for a laparoscopic Nissen fundoplication. When you arrive to interview the patient, you find him sitting up at a 90-degree angle. He states that when he lies flat, he "gets terrible heartburn." What is the risk for this patient in undergoing a general anesthetic? What can you anticipate your anesthesiologist will need?

This patient is at risk for aspiration due to his diagnosis of hiatal hernia and history of esophageal reflux. You can anticipate that your anesthesiologist will perform a rapid sequence induction. You should have the difficult airway equipment available and be prepared to provide cricoid (Sellick maneuver) pressure.

Source: Rothrock, J.C. (Ed.). (2015). *Alexander's Care of the Patient in Surgery* (15th ed., p. 152). St. Louis: Mosby.

Module 3: Incorporate principles of safe positioning — Pages 91-94

Activity — X Marks the Spot

Mark with an "X" the corresponding pressure points associated with the following patient positions. *(See figures on next page.)*

Sources: Rothrock, J.C. (Ed.). (2015). *Alexander's Care of the Patient in Surgery* (15th ed., pp. 174-184). St. Louis: Mosby; Phillips, N. (2013). *Berry and Kohn's Operating Room Technique* (12th ed., pp. 493, 502-508). St. Louis: Mosby.

Activity — Circle the Correct Answer

In the left lateral decubitis position, the patient is lying on the ***LEFT*** side.

When positioning a patient for a Cesarean section, the hip roll is placed under the ***RIGHT*** hip to displace the uterus from the inferior vena cava.

Source: Phillips, N. (2013). *Berry and Kohn's Operating Room Technique*, (12th ed., pp. 507, 713). St. Louis: Mosby.

Activity — X Marks the Spot

Supine

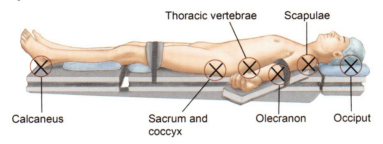

Thoracic vertebrae   Scapulae

Calcaneus   Sacrum and coccyx   Olecranon   Occiput

Prone

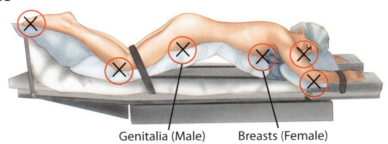

Genitalia (Male)   Breasts (Female)

Lithotomy, boot stirrups

Sitting

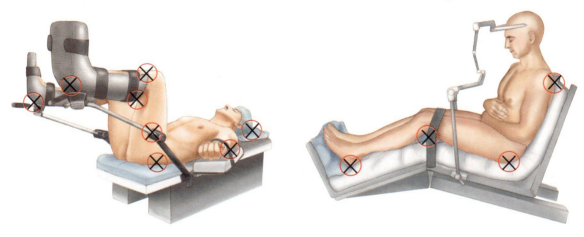

Lateral decubitis

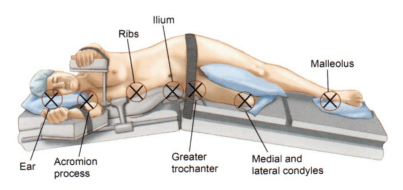

Ribs   Ilium

Malleolus

Ear   Acromion process   Greater trochanter   Medial and lateral condyles

Activity — Matching

Match the position with the associated nerve injury. Answers may be used more than once.

Supine - ***A, E***   A. brachial plexus

Lithotomy - ***B, C***   B.peroneal

Lateral - ***A, B***   C. saphenous

Prone - ***A, E, F***   D. sciatic

Semi-Fowler - ***A***   E. ulnar

Fowler - ***E***   F. radial

> Source: Rothrock, J.C. (Ed.). (2015). *Alexander's Care of the Patient in Surgery* (15th ed., pp. 160-164). St. Louis: Mosby.

Activity — Do You Know?

The preferred placement for the patient's arms in the prone position are ***at the patient's sides.***

> Source: AORN. (2014). Recommended practices for positioning the patient. In *Perioperative Standards and Recommended Practices*, p. 489. Denver: AORN, Inc.

Module 4: Prepare the surgical site — Pages 94-100

Activity — Critical Thinking

You are caring for a patient who is scheduled for reanastomosis of a colostomy. How is the typical skin prep adjusted for this patient?

Surgical preps should normally start at the incision site and move to the periphery. If the incision site is more highly contaminated (e.g., the colostomy) than the surrounding skin, the area with a lower bacterial count should be prepped first. An antiseptic-soaked sponge may be applied to the contaminated area during the prep of the surrounding skin.

> Source: AORN. (2014). Recommended practices for preoperative patient skin antisepsis. In *Perioperative Standards and Recommended Practices*, p. 80. Denver: AORN, Inc.

Case Study Activity

How will Mr. J.'s allergy to shellfish affect the choice of skin antisepsis?

Shellfish allergies are not a contraindication to using iodine-based prep agents.

> Source: AORN. (2014). Recommended practice: Patient skin antisepsis. In *Perioperative Standards and Recommended Practices*, p. 77. Denver: AORN, Inc.

Activity — Color Me

For each illustration, mark the incision (if applicable) and shade the area to be prepped.
See figures below and on following pages.

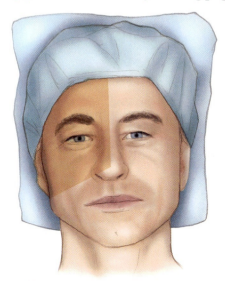

Cataract extraction, right eye

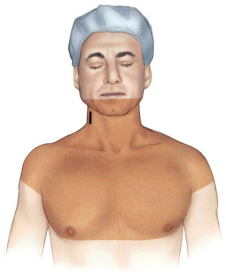

Right carotid endarterectomy

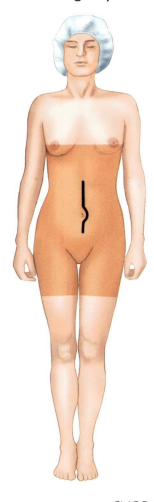

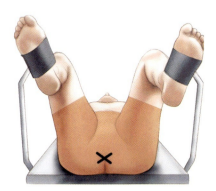

Abdominal/perineal resection

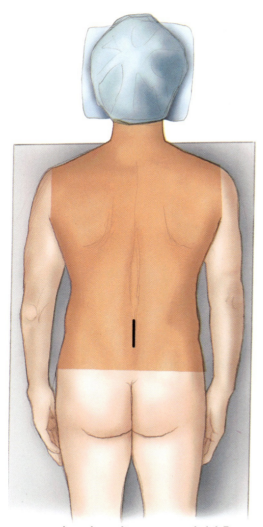

Lumbar discectomy, L4-L5

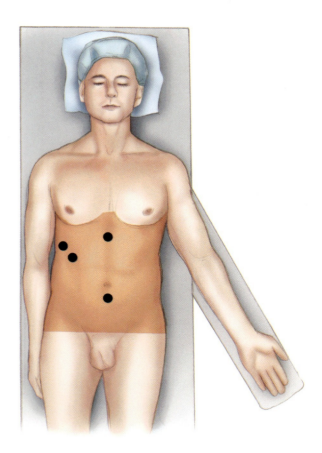

Laparoscopic cholecystectomy

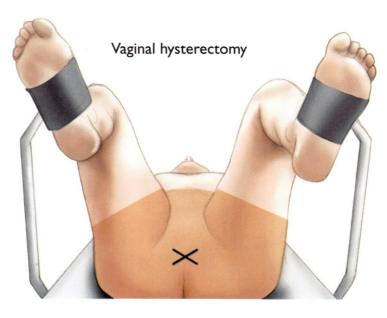

Vaginal hysterectomy

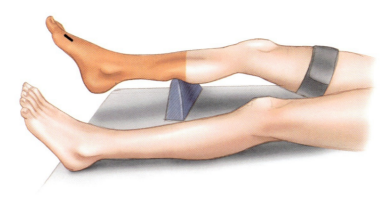

Right bunionectomy

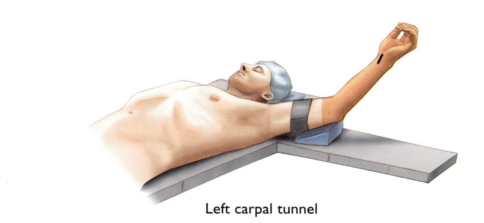

Left carpal tunnel

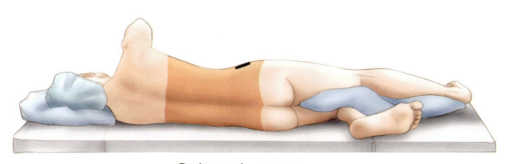

Right nephrectomy

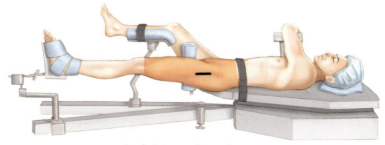

Left hip arthroplasty

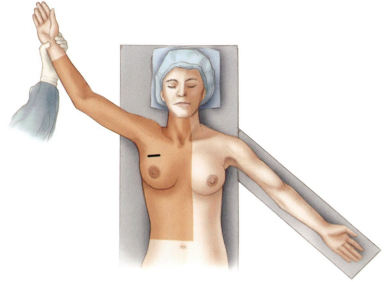

Source: Phillips, N. (2013). *Berry and Kohn's Operating Room Technique* (12th ed., pp. 515-517). St. Louis: Mosby.

Right lumpectomy, right upper quadrant

For the illustrations above and on previous three pages, circle the pictures in which chlorhexidine gluconate may be used as the skin prep agent.

Carotid endarterectomy   *Abdominal prep for abdominal/perineal*
Laparoscopic cholecystectomy   *Right bunionectomy*
Left carpal tunnel   *Right nephrectomy*
Left hip arthroplasty   *Right lumpectomy*
Use with caution for mucous membranes; contraindicated for eye, ear, brain, and spine.

Source: AORN. (2014). Recommended practices for patient skin antisepsis. In *Perioperative Standards and Recommended Practices*, p. 77. Denver: AORN, Inc.

Activity — Critical Thinking

The surgeon requests that hair be removed from the immediate incisional area for an extremely hirsute male scheduled for an inguinal herniorraphy. What is the best method for accomplishing this?

If hair must be removed, it is recommended to be done the day of surgery, in a location outside the OR, with a clipper that is either single-use or with a reusable head that can be disinfected between patients. Only hair that is directly interfering with the surgical procedure should be removed. A razor should not be used as it increases the risk of surgical site infection. A depilatory may be used, but carries with it the increased risk for hypersensitivity reactions.

Source: AORN. (2014). Recommended practices for preoperative patient skin antisepsis. In *Perioperative Standards and Recommended Practices*, pp. 77-78. Denver: AORN, Inc.

Module 5: Apply principles of asepsis — Pages 100-102

Activity — Matching

Match the area with the required appropriate attire. Answers may be used more than once.

Cafeteria: ***E***

Sterile supply room: ***B, C, D***

OR with opened supplies: ***A, B, C, D***

A. mask
B. surgical scrubs
C. hair covering
D. coverall/jumpsuit
E. street clothes

> Source: AORN. (2014). Recommended practices for traffic patterns. In *Perioperative Standards and Recommended Practices*, p. 119. Denver: AORN, Inc.

Activity — Fill In the Blank

For the following procedures, write in the corresponding wound classification:

Total knee replacement: ***Clean wound, Class I***
Incision and drainage of abscess, status postop posterior spinal fusion: ***Dirty/infected wound, Class IV***
Appendectomy, unruptured: ***Clean/Contaminated wound, Class II***
Open reduction internal fixation open fracture right radius/ulna: ***Contaminated wound, Class III***
Gunshot wound to abdomen: ***Contaminated wound, Class III***
Bowel resection, no spillage: ***Clean contaminated, Class II***
Rhytidectomy: ***Clean wound, Class I***
Bowel resection, spillage: ***Contaminated wound, Class III***
Myringotomy: ***Contaminated wound, Class III if signs of infection***

> Source: Rothrock, J.C. (Ed.). (2015). *Alexander's Care of the Patient in Surgery* (15th ed., pp. 258-259). St. Louis: Mosby.

Activity — Critical Thinking

Circle the most effective method for disinfecting hands after caring for a patient with *Clostridium difficile.*

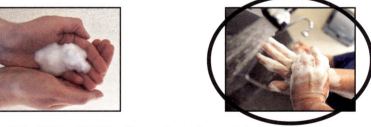

> Source: Rothrock, J.C. (Ed.). (2015). *Alexander's Care of the Patient in Surgery* (15th ed., p. 72). St. Louis: Mosby.

Activity — Short Answer

1. While turning over your room, you drop an unopened box of 4X4 radiopaque sponges on the floor. What is the correct action?

Any time the sterility of an item is in question, it should not be used.

    Source: Rothrock, J.C. (Ed.). (2015). *Alexander's Care of the Patient in Surgery* (15th ed., p. 103). St. Louis: Mosby

2. You are scrubbed for a laparoscopic cholecystectomy. The surgeon asks you to move to the other side of the table to hold the camera while initiating an additional port site. What is the appropriate way to pass the other scrubbed members of the team?

Members should pass face-to-face or back-to-back while maintaining safe distances from the sterile field.

    Source: AORN. (2014). Recommended practices for maintaining a sterile field. In *Perioperative Standards and Recommended Practices*, p. 108. Denver: AORN, Inc.

3. After opening up and counting your sterile field for a laparoscopic-assisted vaginal hysterectomy (LAVH), the charge nurse informs you that your surgeon has an emergency in labor and delivery. Your scrub technician asks if the back table can be covered. What is the correct response?

When there is an unanticipated delay, the sterile field that has been prepared and will not be used immediately may be covered with sterile drapes. The drapes should be applied and removed in a way that will not contaminate the contents of the sterile field. The sterile field should not be left unattended.

    Source: AORN. (2014). Recommended practices for sterile technique. In *Perioperative Standards and Recommended Practices*, pp. 105-106. Denver: AORN, Inc.

Module 6: Provide perioperative nursing care during operative and invasive procedures — Pages 103-105

"Go To" Case Study Activity

From your previously developed concept map and the patient assessment, develop a plan of care for the intraoperative component of Mr. J.'s perioperative experience.

1. Identify the intraoperative nursing interventions that will need to be implemented for Mr. J.s' surgical procedure. Some of these are typical for every surgery (e.g., infection prevention, principles of aseptic technique, skin antisepsis), while others will be specific for Mr. J. *(See sample answers in the Study Guide Toolbox at http://www.cc-institute.org/toolbox)*

2. Arrange the intraoperative activities from your list under their corresponding "major problems" boxes you developed in Chapters 1 and 2. *(See sample answers in the Toolbox at http://www.cc-institute.org/toolbox)*

3. At what pressure should the tourniquet be set?

Standard setting is 300-350 mmHg for lower limbs. A lower setting may be used by utilizing a safety margin of 40-80 mmHg based on the limb occlusion pressure.

Source: AORN. (2014). Recommended practices for pneumatic tourniqet. In *Perioperative Standards and Recommended Practices*, pp. 192-193. Denver: AORN, Inc.

4. Where should the electrosurgical dispersive electrode pad be placed?

The electrosurgical dispersive electrode pad should not be placed over a metal implant (in this case, Mr. J.'s right hip). It should be placed as close to the surgical site as possible, e.g, the left flank.

Source: AORN. (2014). Recommended practices for electrosurgery. In *Perioperative Standards and Recommended Practices*, pp. 128-129. Denver: AORN, Inc.

Activity — Short Answer

A 17-year-old patient returns to your facility seven months postoperatively for removal of an infected Harrington rod implant. The wound cultures *Staphylococcus aureus*. Is this considered a surgical site infection? Why or why not?

In January 2014 the CDC changed the reporting period for SSI in spinal fusions to 90 days. Based on the new guidelines, this would not be classified as a SSI by the CDC for reporting.

Source: CDC. (2014, Jan.). Surgical Site Infection (SSI) Event, pp. 9-14. Retrieved Feb. 28, 2014, from http://www.cdc.gov/nhsn/pdfs/pscmanual/9pscssicurrent.pdf

Activity — Name That Incision

Name the abdominal incisions in the diagram.

Source: Rothrock, J.C. (Ed.). (2015). *Alexander's Care of the Patient in Surgery* (15th ed., p. 306). St. Louis: Mosby.

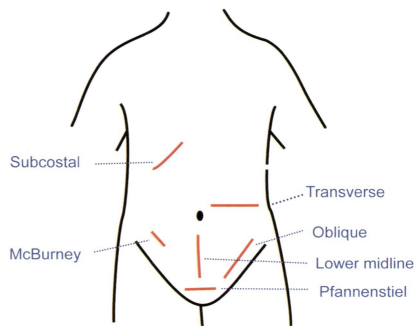

Subcostal

Transverse

Oblique

McBurney

Lower midline

Pfannenstiel

Activity — Matching

Match the incision types shown in the illustration on page 135 to their corresponding surgical procedure. Use each answer only once.

Lower midline: *C*
Oblique: *D*
Pfannenstiel: *A*
Subcostal: *E*
McBurney: *B*
Transverse: *F*

A. abdominal hysterectomy
B. appendectomy
C. radical retropubic prostatectomy
D. open inguinal herniorraphy
E. hepatic resection
F. choledochojejunostomy

Source: Phillips, N. (2013). *Berry and Kohn's Operating Room Technique* (12th ed., pp. 547-550). St. Louis: Mosby.

Activity — Short Answer

Your patient is scheduled for an ulnar nerve release, left elbow; he states that he has an implantable cardiodefibrillator. What is the safest electrosurgical method to use, and why?

The bipolar ESU provides hemostasis at the surgical site with less potential stimulation of adjacent tissue. Because the active and return electrodes are contained in the tips of the instrument, the current passes between the two poles and only affects the tissue between the poles. There is less chance of stray or alternate pathways with this form of electrocautery. Bipolar electrosurgery uses a lower voltage so that there is less potential for electromagnetic interference.

Sources: AORN. (2014). Recommended practices for electrosurgery. In *Perioperative Standards and Recommended Practices*, p. 131. Denver: AORN, Inc.; Phillips, N. (2013). *Berry and Kohn's Operating Room Technique* (12th ed., p. 354). St. Louis: Mosby.

Module 7: Identify and control environmental factors — Pages 106-108

Activity — Fill in the Blank

For each of the following environmental controls, list the acceptable parameters:

Air exchanges: OR: ***minimum 15/hour, recommended 20-25;*** Cardiac cath lab: ***15/hour;*** Sterile storage area: ***4/hour;*** Decontamination area: ***at least 6/hour***

Humidity: OR: ***30-60%;*** Cardiac cath lab: ***30-60%;*** Decontamination area: ***20-60%***

Temperature: OR: ***68°F-73°F;*** Cardiac cath lab: ***70°F-75°F;*** Decontamination area: ***60°F-65°F***

Air pressure in the OR should be ***greater*** than the surrounding corridors.

Source: AORN. (2014). Recommended practices for: Minimally invasive surgery, p. 159; Sterilization, p. 578. In *Perioperative Standards and Recommended Practices*. Denver: AORN, Inc; Rothrock, J.C. (Ed.). (2015). *Alexander's Care of the Patient in Surgery* (15th ed., p. 87). St. Louis: Mosby.

Activity — Short Answer

For each source of noise, list a nursing intervention to reduce its risk of disrupting the environment and impacting patient safety:

Examples of interventions include the following (you may think of others).

Beeper/pager/cell phone: *Place on silent whenever possible.*

Monitor alarms: *Turn to the lowest setting that is still audible.*

Electronic music devices (radios, CD players): *Turn to the lowest setting that is still audible. Requests to turn off distracting music should be honored.*

Overhead pages and announcements: *Use text paging.*

Telephones: *Limit conversations to brief communication. Practice telephone etiquette when answering the phone.*

Staff communication:
Minimize the number of people present during procedures and limit traffic flow.
Establish and enforce times when noise levels should be routinely be reduced (e.g., induction, emergence, counts).
Use a low speaking voice, and remind others to do the same.
Increase staff awareness via education.
Post signs to remind staff to keep noise levels low.
Minimize irrelevant conversation.

Sources: Rothrock, J.C. (Ed.). (2015). *Alexander's Care of the Patient in Surgery* (15th ed., p. 125). St. Louis: Mosby; AORN. (2009). Position statement on noise in the perioperative setting. Retrieved March 1, 2014, from http://www.aorn.org/Clinical_Practice/Position_Statements/Position_Statements.aspx

Case Study Activity

As the anesthesia care provider hands you a tube of blood for a blood chemistry analysis for Mr. J., it slips out of your hand and drops to the floor, breaking the tube. What is the best way to clean up the spill?

Gloves must be worn; the broken tube should be placed in the sharps container. The blood should be removed with an absorbent material, and the area disinfected with an EPA-registered disinfectant as soon as possible. The contaminated cleaning cloth should be placed in a designated labeled or color-coded receptacle. The gloves used during cleaning the spill should be removed, and hand hygiene performed.

Source: AORN. (2014). Recommended practices for environmental cleaning in the perioperative setting. In *Perioperative Standards and Recommended Practices*, p. 266. Denver: AORN, Inc.

Activity — Critical Thinking

How does end of procedure (turnover) cleaning between cases differ from that done at the end of the day (terminal cleaning)?

End of procedure cleaning is performed between surgical procedures. It includes, but is not limited to, all horizontal surfaces, surgical lights, the OR bed, non-disposable positioning devices, patient transport vehicles, all receptables (e.g., bins, kick buckets, pails), and high touch surfaces if applicable. Additional cleaning may be needed for areas that are soiled or potentially soiled by splash, splatter, or spray of infected materials.

Terminal cleaning is performed in ORs and scrub/utility areas at the end of the daily schedule. All exposed surfaces should be cleaned, including surgical lights; external lighting tracks; fixed and ceiling-mounted equipment; all furniture, including wheels and casters; equipment (e.g., electrosurgical units, suction canister holders); handles of cabinets and push plates; ventilation face plates; horizontal surfaces; the entire floor (either via wet vacuum or single-use mop); the entire OR bed, including the underside of mattress and the metal frame of OR bed; kick buckets; and scrub sinks.

Source: AORN. (2014). Recommended practices for environmental cleaning. In *Perioperative Standards and Recommended Practices*, pp. 260-264. Denver: AORN, Inc.; Rothrock, J. C. (Ed.). (2015). *Alexander's Care of the Patient in Surgery* (15th ed., pp. 120-121). St. Louis: Mosby.

Module 8: Monitor and intervene to reduce the risk of complications and adverse outcomes — Pages 108-111

Activity — Fill in the Blank

The three principles related to radiation protection are: *time, distance, and shielding*.

Sources: AORN. (2014). Recommended practices for reducing radiological exposure. In *Perioperative Standards and Recommended Practices*, p. 321. Denver: AORN, Inc.; Rothrock, J.C. (Ed.). (2015). *Alexander's Care of the Patient in Surgery* (15th ed., p. 64). St. Louis: Mosby.

Activity — Critical Thinking

1. You are the circulating nurse for an 11-year-old boy undergoing an open reduction internal fixation for a right malleolar fracture from a skate-board accident. You notice that the tourniquet time is approaching 60 minutes. What action, if any, needs to be taken?

It is recommended that tourniquet time not exceed 75 minutes for lower extremities for pediatric patients. The surgeon should be notified of the tourniquet time and, based on the length of time remaining to complete the surgery, collaborate with the anesthesia provider on releasing the tourniquet and reperfusing the limb.

Source: AORN. (2014). Recommended practices for the use of the pneumatic tourniquet in perioperative practice. In *Perioperative Standards and Recommended Practices*, p. 194. Denver: AORN, Inc.

2. Your patient is scheduled for a laser tonsillectomy. What safety mechanisms should be in place to care for your patient?

Sample Answers (responses may vary but should include):
- *Identify that a laser will be in use by posting a warning sign on OR door. Doors should remain closed.*
- *Cover windows with a barrier that blocks transmission of the laser beam as appropriate.*
- *Check laser for appropriate functioning according to manufacturer's recommendations.*
- *Designate a laser assistant who has no other responsibilities.*
- *Reflective surfaces should be minimized. Use the appropriate instruments. Cover reflective surfaces and exposed tissue with saline-saturated sponges.*
- *Patient and staff should wear appropriate eye protection.*
- *Surgical smoke plume should be evacuated.*
- *The risk of fire should be mitigated by employing the appropriate fire safety mechanisms.*
- *A laser-resistant endotracheal tube should be provided for anesthesia. Saline with dye should be used to fill the balloon to facilitate detection of a puncture. Moistened packs should be placed on each side of tube.*

Source: AORN. (2014). Recommended practices for laser safety. In *Perioperative Standards and Recommended Practices*, pp. 143-149. Denver: AORN, Inc.

Activity — Critical Thinking

What interventions can be implemented to safely transfer a patient scheduled for a laparascopic Roux-en-Y gastric bypass procedure?

Patients should be encouraged to move themselves whenever possible. Consider using a mechanical or air lateral transfer device if available. The destination surface should be slightly lower for all lateral moves. A minimum of four caregivers will be needed to transfer a patient. These resources should be available prior to the move to expedite OR time. Consider placing a patient in a patient bed (not a gurney) for transfer to PACU postoperatively.

Source: AORN. (2014). Guidance statement: Safe patient handling and movement in the perioperative setting. In *Perioperative Standards and Recommended Practices*, p. 618. Denver: AORN, Inc.

Case Study Activity

1. Dr. S. repeatedly asks for the coagulation power on the electrosurgical unit to be increased. What steps should be taken in trouble-shooting a possible problem?

- *Confirm power settings with surgeon; communicate what "normal" settings are based on manufacturer's recommendations.*
- *Check patient return electrode to make certain it is in good contact with the patient.*
- *Check all connections (patient return electrode, electrode cord, and power cord) to ensure that they are plugged in correctly.*
- *Check for presence of an alternate ground (EKG electrode, Mr. J.'s body in contact with metal on the bed or the positioning device).*
- *Replace patient return electrode if necessary; if problem continues, remove electrosurgical unit from service. Send patient return electrode and unit to the biomedical department for evaluation.*
- *Carefully assess Mr. J. for undetected thermal injuries.*

Source: AORN. (2014). Recommended practices for electrosurgery. In *Perioperative Standards and Recommended Practices*, pp. 124-125. Denver: AORN, Inc.

2. Upon completion of the surgery, a slightly reddened area is noted under the site for Mr. J.'s electrosurgical dispersive electrode pad. What steps need to be taken in treating and reporting this incident?

Sample responses; yours may vary:
Note that the variance report example below contains more specific details than the patient record. The fact that an occurrence/variance form was completed should NOT be documented in the patient's permanent record.

- *Patient record: "Patient dispersive electrode removed at end of procedure. Reddened area noted under electrode approximately 2 inches by 3 inches at the distal end of dispersive electrode site. Dr. Smith notified. Silvadene cream applied per his order."*
- *Variance report: "Patient dispersive electrode removed at end of procedure. Reddened area noted under pad area approximately 2 inches by 3 inches at the distal end of dispersive electrode site. Dr. Smith notified. Electrosurgery unit #5 removed from service and sent to biomedical department for evaluation, along with grounding pad, serial number 453S2. All other grounding pads with same serial number removed from stock and quarantined."*

Source: Phillips, N. (2013). *Berry and Kohn's Operating Room Technique* (12th ed., p. 50). St. Louis: Mosby.

Module 9: Prepare and label specimens — Pages 111-112

Activity — Short Answer

Identification of the specimen should be confirmed verbally between the circulating nurse and the surgeon using a "read back" communication similar to that used with verbal orders. What information needs to be communicated between the surgeon and circulating nurse?

Originating source of specimen (e.g., right or left, site)
Type of tissue
Clinical diagnosis
Any pertinent information (e.g., patient history, suture marking for orientation, requests for tests)

Source: AORN. (2014). Recommended practices for specimen care and handling. In *Perioperative Standards and Recommended Practices*, p. 377. Denver: AORN, Inc.

Activity — True or False

1. As long as an instrument is used to transfer the specimen from the sterile field to the specimen jar, the circulator is not required to wear gloves or eye protection.

False. Standard precautions should be used at all times when handling specimens.

Source: Rothrock, J.C. (Ed.). (2015). *Alexander's Care of the Patient in Surgery* (15th ed., p. 32). St. Louis: Mosby.

2. The specimen label should be placed on the lid of the container.

False; the label should be placed on the container.

> Source: AORN. (2014). Recommended practices for specimen care and handling. In *Periopera-tive Standards and Recommended Practices*, p. 377. Denver: AORN, Inc.

Module 10: Perform counts — Pages 113-115

Activity — Do You Know?

How many strategies can you list to help prevent a retained surgical item?

Sample responses:
Avoid unnecessary distractions/talking, which interfere with clear communication between circulator and scrub person.
Immediately document items added to the count.
Account for counted items that have fallen/been removed from the sterile field.
Perform counts consistently in a standardized manner to minimize chance for error.
Keep sterile field organized.
Confine sharps to a designated area.
Use only radiopaque items in the wound.
Report discrepancies in count immediately.
Verify items concurrently.

> Source: AORN. (2014). Recommended practices for prevention of retained surgical items. In *Perioperative Standards and Recommended Practices*, p. 334. Denver: AORN, Inc.

Activity — Critical Thinking

You are counting sponges with the scrub person in preparation for an abdominal hysterectomy. The package of 4X4 radiopaque sponges you have opened contains 9 sponges instead of 10. What should you do?

Packages containing an incorrect number of radiopaque sponges should be removed from the room before the patient arrives to decrease confusion and minimize the likelihood for error.

> Source: AORN. (2014). Recommended practices for prevention of retained surgical items. In *Perioperative Standards and Recommended Practices*, p. 336. Denver: AORN, Inc.

Activity — Scramble

Number the following steps in the correct order for completing a sponge and suture count.

1. Before the procedure
2. Before closure of a cavity (e.g., uterus or bladder) within a cavity
3. When wound (peritoneum) closure begins
4. At skin closure

List three other circumstances when a count should be performed:

1. Whenever new items are added
2. At the time of permanent relief of either scrub person or circulator
3. At the request of any member of the perioperative team.

Source: AORN. (2014). Recommended practices for prevention of retained surgical items. In *Perioperative Standards and Recommended Practices*, pp. 334, 336, 338. Denver: AORN, Inc.

Case Study Activity

Mr. J.'s surgery is near completion. As a needle holder and needle were returned to the scrub person, he noted that the needle was bent with the tip of the needle missing. Explain your immediate course of action to prevent a retained surgical item. How would you document these issues and the patient care you provided?

The circulator must notify the surgeon immediately of the missing piece of needle so that the surgeon can do a methodical wound search to look for the item. The sterile field, Mayo stand, back table, floor, kick bucket, and discarded items must be searched. If the item is found and retrieved, then the count can be documented as correct. If the surgeon and scrub nurse cannot find the needle tip, then an x-ray must be ordered. The x-ray should be read by a radiologist and a report sent to the operating room. If the needle tip is not recovered, then the count must be documented as incorrect, the results of the x-ray must be documented, and an occurrence or variance report must be completed. The surgeon should remain in the OR until the needle is either found or it is determined with certainty that it is not in the wound.

Sources: AORN. (2014). Recommended practices for prevention of retained surgical items. In *Perioperative Standards and Recommended Practices*, pp. 341, 343-344. Denver: AORN, Inc.; AORN. (2011). *Perioperative Nursing Data Set* (PNDS). (3rd ed., pp. 146-149). Denver: AORN, Inc.; Rothrock, J.C. (Ed.). (2015). *Alexander's Care of the Patient in Surgery* (15th ed., p. 32). St. Louis: Mosby.

Module 11: Maintain accurate patient records — Pages 116-117

Activity — Critical Thinking

You work in a free-standing ambulatory surgery center that enjoys a thriving plastic surgery practice. Your facility has just received a letter from the FDA recalling a certain brand of breast implant. What information from the patients' records do you need to have in determining which of your patients are affected by this recall?

Name and contact information of patient
Name and contact information of the surgeon
Name of manufacturer/distributor
Lot, model, and serial numbers
Type and size of implant
Location the device was implanted
Manufacturer or expiration date as appropriate
Any other information as requested by the FDA

Source: Rothrock, J.C. (Ed.). (2015). *Alexander's Care of the Patient in Surgery* (15th ed., p. 830). St. Louis: Mosby.

CHAPTER 4:
Communication

> ### Test Specifications:
> ### 9% of CNOR test questions are based on Communication.

Introduction

Have you ever gone past a piece of equipment in the hall with a sign taped to it that says "Broken"? Although this information is useful in determining that it shouldn't be used, there is no guidance related to who is responsible for repairs or the exact nature of the problem. Extra time and effort is expended to track down and recover the information needed to actually get the equipment repaired and back in service. If the information obtained is inaccurate or incomplete, there's a good chance that the repair may not be done correctly, if at all.

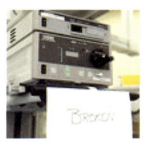

Miscommunication is not limited to equipment repairs. The leading cause of reported sentinel events (those that cause death or serious injury) in the OR is communication breakdown (Johnson, et al, 2013).

Perioperative patient care is delivered by an interdisciplinary team of health care practitioners, with no single member of the team having the knowledge to develop a comprehensive plan of care without input from other members of the team. It is through communication that we access knowledge about our patients and interact with our colleagues. Each person who interacts with the patient gathers information to support his or her clinical perspective. Creating a practice environment that fosters a culture of safety and positive outcomes for patients requires the knowledge and use of of effective communication skills.

This chapter will help you to apply communication strategies to a variety of learning activities. Clinical scenarios and case studies provide opportunities to identify, prioritize, and transmit information that will promote safe patient care.

Module 1: Verbal and Nonverbal Communication

Delivering the best care possible requires the perioperative nurse to solicit input from others and to communicate consistently, clearly, and assertively. The perioperative setting is unique in that decisions are often communicated quickly, under stressful and noisy conditions, with limited facial visual clues, and with serious ramifications if an error is made in either the transmission or receipt of the message. Listening is especially important in a hectic environment such as the OR.

Safe nursing care depends on nurses who can communicate effectively. "Reading back" has been found to be a useful way to verify what has been heard (e.g., "lobe" vs. "node" when receiving a specimen from the field).

Competency Outcomes

To successfully complete the activities in this module, you will need to be able to:

1. Identify effective communication strategies to promote quality patient outcomes.
2. Implement standardized communication processes.

Recommended Readings

Alexander's Care of the Patient in Surgery. (2015, 15th ed.), Chapter 1: Concepts basic to perioperative nursing; Chapter 2: Patient safety and risk management.

AORN. (2011). Position statement: Creating a practice environment of safety. Retrieved Feb. 21, 2014, from http://www.aorn.org/Clinical_Practice/Position_Statements/ Position_Statements.aspx

Berry and Kohn's Operating Room Technique. (2013, 12th ed.), Chapter 6: Administration of perioperative patient care services; Chapter 7: The patient: The reason for your existence; Chapter 21: Preoperative preparation of the patient.

Perioperative Standards and Recommended Practices. (2014), Recommended practices: Transfer of patient care information.

Key Words

Communication, culture of safety, hand-off, never event, read back, SBAR, standardized communication plan, Universal Protocol, WHO checklist

Activity — Short Answer

Closed-ended (directive) questions are answered using "yes" or "no." An open-ended or non-directive question offers an opportunity to expand on the answer.

For each closed-ended (directive) preoperative interview question listed on the following page, provide an associated open-ended (non-directive) question. Compare the differences in quality and quantity of information received utilizing both approaches.

1. Have you had anything to eat or drink in the past eight hours?

2. Is your name John?

3. Are you undergoing an appendectomy today?

4. Do you need any other help today?

Case Study Activity

1. What parts of Mr. J.'s assessment requires an immediate intervention?

2. Use the SBAR (Situation, Background, Assessment, Recommendation) format to communicate this information to the surgeon and anesthesia care provider.

Activity — Critical Thinking

A 38-year-old female was admitted to the OR for a scheduled left L3-L4 decompression laminectomy. The consent was confirmed, and correct side and level were verified verbally and marked with the patient's participation in the preoperative area by the preoperative nurse. X-ray images were with the patient and placed on the viewer in the assigned OR. The OR was set up for a left-sided laminectomy with the electrosurgery unit (ESU) and bipolar cautery pedals placed on the floor according to the physician's preference card for a left-sided laminectomy. The patient was anesthetized, intubated, placed in the prone position, prepped, and draped by the surgical assistant before the surgeon's arrival in the OR.

The surgeon reviewed the x-rays on the viewer, and abruptly requested that the nurse move the ESU and bipolar cautery pedals to the other side. The nurse did not question his request for the change or re-verify the x-rays, but repositioned the pedals accordingly. The nurse was out of the room retrieving sutures during the time-out, but the surgeon verified the site and side with the anesthesiologist, and the surgery began on time.

The circulating nurse documented that the time-out had occurred and that all components of the Universal Protocol had been met after verifying the information directly with the anesthesiologist.

At the conclusion of the procedure, the physician reviewed the postoperative x-rays, history and physical exam findings, and consent forms only to realize he had operated on the wrong side. The patient was taken to recovery, where she was informed of the wrong-side surgery. She was returned to the OR for a second procedure.

1. Highlight the areas in the scenario above in which breaks in communication or protocol influenced patient outcomes.

2. For each highlighted area, provide an example of "speaking up" that may have helped avert the occurrence.

3. What should be done to prevent the above situation from reoccurring in the future?

Activity — Critical Thinking

As she leaves the room to get additional suture, the circulating nurse asks the student she is precepting to put sterile saline in the basin opened on the ring stand. When she returns, she sees an unopened bottle of sterile saline sitting in the basin. How could this break in technique have been avoided?

"Go To" Activity — Check It Out!

Go to Question #13, Healthy work environment, under the Perioperative question of the week tab in the Study Guide Toolbox at http://www.cc-institute.org/toolbox for an additional critical-thinking activity related to communication in the workplace.

"Go To" Activity — Skill Building

Review the Universal Protocol and WHO checklists. How do they differ? How does your facility's perioperative safety checklist compare with these two documents?

Additional Readings/Resources

Agency for Healthcare Research and Quality. (n.d.). Never Events. Retrieved Feb. 21, 2014, from http://psnet.ahrq.gov/primer.aspx?primerID=3

AORN. (2013). Patient Hand Off Tool Kit. Retrieved Feb. 20, 2014, from http://www.aorn.org/PracticeResources/ToolKits/PatientHandOffToolKit/

AORN, Vitalsmarts, & AACN. The Silent Treatment: Why safety tools and checklists aren't enough to save lives. Retrieved Feb. 21, 2014, from http://silenttreatmentstudy.com/

Clark, G.J. (2013). Strategies for preventing distractions and interruptions in the OR. *AORN Journal, (97)*6, 702-707.

Cyetic, E. (2011). Communication in the perioperative setting. *AORN Journal, (94)*3, 261-270.

Gawande, A. (2010). *The Checklist Manifesto.* New York, NY: Henry Holt and Co.

Gillespie, B.M., Chaboyer, W., & Fairweather, N. (2012). Interruptions and miscommunications in surgery: An observational study. *AORN Journal, (95)*5, 576-590.

Gillespie, B.M., Chaboyer, W., & Murray, P. (2010). Enhancing communication in surgery through team training interventions: A systematic literature review. *AORN Journal, (92)*6, 642-657.

Johnson, H.L., & Kimsey, D. (2012). Patient safety: Break the silence. *AORN Journal, (95)*5, 591-601.

Mitchell, E.N. (2013). Improving communication and building trust. *AORN Journal, (98)*3, 218-219.

The Joint Commission. (2014). Facts About the Universal Protocol. Retrieved Feb. 21, 2014, from http://www.jointcommission.org/standards_information/up.aspx

The Joint Commision. (2014). National Patient Safety Goals. UP.01.01.01: Conduct a preprocedure verification process; UP.01.02.01: Mark the procedure site; UP.01.03.01: A time-out is performed. Retrieved Feb. 21, 2014, from http://www.jointcommission.org/hap_2014_npsgs/

Wahr, J.A., Prager, R.L., Abernathy, J.H., et al. (2013). Patient Safety in the Cardiac Operating Room: Human factors and teamwork: A scientific statement from the American Heart Association. doi: 10.1161/CIR.ObO13e3182a38efa. Retrieved Feb 21, 2014, from http://circ.ahajournals.org/content/128/10/1139

Watson, D.S. (2009). Implementing the Universal Protocol. *AORN Journal, 90*(2), 283-287.

World Health Organization (WHO). (2014). Safe Surgery Saves Lives. Retrieved Feb. 21, 2014, from http://www.who.int/patientsafety/safesurgery/en/

Module 2: Written Communication

Written documentation, either a physical chart or an electronic record, should provide consistent, accessible information, and as such is a prime communication tool for managing patient care safely and effectively among multidisciplinary health care providers. Documentation must be clear, concise, objective, and complete, because multidisciplinary caregivers rely heavily on written communication in making patient care decisions.

Nurses learn very early that "if it wasn't documented, it wasn't done!" Observations and patient interventions that are not documented are unavailable to other team members to help with decision making related to patient care. Because accurate information is integral to planning appropriate patient care, failing to document, documenting poorly, or documenting incorrectly are all serious errors with a significant impact on patient outcomes.

Remember — the chart is a legal document. Unexpected events often trigger an investigation, and it will be very difficult for you to remember the details months or years afterward. Having comprehensive documentation of the facts is essential for performance improvement audits, perioperative nursing research, and risk mitigation.

Competency Outcomes

To successfully complete the activities in this module, you will need to be able to:

1. Describe best practices in written communication that promote quality patient care outcomes.
2. Identify regulatory influences on written communication in the health care setting.
3. Discuss the legal implications of written documentation.

Recommended Reading

Alexander's Care of the Patient in Surgery. (2015, 15th ed.), Chapter 2: Patient safety and risk management.

AORN. (2011). Position statement: Creating a practice environment of safety. Retrieved Feb. 21, 2014, from http://www.aorn.org/Clinical_Practice/Position_Statements/Position_Statements.aspx

Berry and Kohn's Operating Room Technique. (2013, 12th ed.), Chapter 2: Foundations of perioperative patient care standards; Chapter 3: Legal, regulatory, and ethical issues; Chapter 6: Administration of perioperative patient care services; Chapter 7: The patient: The reason for your existence; Chapter 21: Preoperative preparation of the patient.

Perioperative Standards and Recommended Practices. (2014),
• Recommended practices for perioperative health care information management.
• Recommended practices for transfer of patient care information.

Key Words

Communication, documentation, HIPAA, National Patient Safety Goals, PNDS, regulatory agency, standardized communication tool, surgical safety checklist, The Joint Commission, WHO checklist

Activity — Search and Circle

According to the Health Insurance Portability and Accountability Act (HIPAA), personal health information includes:
- Name
- Address
- Birthdate
- Social security number
- Phone number, e-mail, fax
- Past, present, or future physical or mental health condition

Please circle the items on the schedule board that violate HIPAA regulations.

Time	Room	Patient	Dr.	Procedure/ Anesth
0730–0900	OR1	J. Brown SS# 100-98-0004	Smith	Laparoscopic cholecystectomy / General
0915–1145	OR1	J. Brown SS# 999-00-1234	Smith	Right carotid endarterectomy/General
1200–1330	OR1	Carl Johnson Patient is HIV +	Smith	Right inguinal hernia repair/Moderate Sedation
0730–0815	OR2	T. Adams Call his mom at 719-800-1623 when he's in PACU	Brats	Tonsillectomy/General
0730–0900	OR3	Shirley Nickle – e-mail postoperative instructions to smick@yahoo.org	Short	Abdominal hysterectomy /General
0915–1045	OR#3	Carol D. DOB 07/08/56	Short	Abdominal hysterectomy /General

Activity — Critical Thinking

A patient is scheduled for an exploratory laparotomy for a possible perforated viscus. When you arrive to interview the patient, you find the patient confused about the scheduled surgical procedure and he asks to speak to the surgeon. The permit has been signed, but the surgeon is not immediately available. What is the most appropriate course of action?

Case Study Activity

You document in Mr. J.'s electronic medical record that an incident report (occurrence report) has been completed related to an incorrect suture count. From a legal standpoint, what are the ramifications of this documentation?

"Go To" Activity — Skill Building

Organizational policy should clearly identify appropriate communication strategies to be followed in sharing confidential patient information with designated family or friends by phone, in public waiting areas, and in any phase of the perioperative process. Review how your facility releases information on patient status to family members. Compare current practice to HIPAA privacy rules, found at http://www.hhs.gov/ocr/privacy/hipaa/understanding/summary/

Additional Readings/Resources

AORN. (2011). *Perioperative Nursing Data Set* (3rd ed.). Denver: AORN, Inc.

Beach, M.J., & Sions, J.A. (2011). Surviving OR computerization. *AORN Journal, (93)*2, 226-241.

Brusco, J.M. (2011). Trending towards paperless. *AORN Journal, (94)*1, 13-18.

Centers for Medicare and Medicaid Services (CMS). (2012). The HIPAA Law and Related Information. Retrieved March 24, 2014, from http://www.cms.gov/Regulations-and-Guidance/HIPAA-Administrative-Simplification/HIPAAGenInfo/TheHIPAALawand Related-Information.html

Giarrizzo-Wilson, S. (2009). Using AORN's standardized data framework for documentation. *AORN Journal, (90)*6, 919-920.

Stanton, C. (2010). Implementing health IT. *AORN Journal, (92)*6, S81-S83.

Stanton, C. (2011). Connections: Managing health information. *AORN Journal, (94)*2, C1.

Styer, K.A., Ashley, S.W., Schmidt, I., et al. (2011). Implementing the World Health Organization Surgical Safety Checklist: A model for future perioperative initiatives. *AORN Journal, 94*(6), 590-598.

Sweeney, P. (2010). The effects of information technology on perioperative nursing. *AORN Journal,* (92)5, 528-543.

U.S. Dept. of Health and Human Services (HHS). Health Information Privacy. Retrieved Feb. 21, 2014, from http://www.hhs.gov/ocr/privacy/index.html

Chapter Summary

Communication is an essential component of multidisciplinary practice. The effectiveness of each professional's decisions and interventions depends on the information he or she has received. Clear, consistent, and comprehensive communication with the patient, family, and all members of the multidisciplinary team facilitates patient safety and optimal outcomes.

As patient advocates, perioperative registered nurses have a duty to protect the patient from injury and to safeguard the patient's health, welfare, and safety. Effective communication, reporting, documentation, and compliance with established standards of practice and hospital policies can support advocacy and help ensure patient safety.

Glossary

Accountable — The state of being answerable to self, patient, profession, and agency for nursing care given.

Advance directive — A patient's signed and witnessed directive regarding health care, life-sustaining, and end-of-life decisions.

American Nurses Association (ANA) — Professional organization representing registered nurses. The ANA promulgates the Code of Ethics for nurses with interpretive statements that articulates the moral commitment to maintain the values and ethical obligations of all nurses. (www.ana.org)

Assessment — Assessment begins with data collection and ends with the formation of nursing diagnoses. It includes patient's history and physical exam findings, vital signs, and all aspects of presenting condition. Assessment is ongoing during the perioperative period (i.e., includes preoperative, intraoperative, postoperative).

Autonomy — In the context of health care, autonomy is the patient's self-determination or ability and power to make his or her own decisions regarding health care.

Communication — The transfer of information that requires a sender, a message, and a receiver. Transmission may be verbal, non-verbal, or written.

Continuum of care — Care of patients undergoing operative or other invasive procedures is planned and implemented along a continuum — from the time the decision to undergo surgery is made, through the intraoperative period, and for an undetermined postoperative period until the patient's health status is improved or a specified health goal is reached.

Culture of patient safety — An atmosphere of mutual trust in which all staff members can talk freely about safety issues and how to solve them without fear of blame or punishment. It is considered essential to the improvement of patient safety in any organization.

Demonstration and return demonstration — The act of teaching that involves the visible, active demonstration of an activity, then involving the learner by having him or her demonstrate the identical activity back to the teacher.

Discharge planning — The process of assessing the needs of patients for post-procedure care; developing a coordinated and multidisciplinary plan to provide the care required (including patient and family education, available services, and referral agencies and support groups); and evaluating the plan. The process begins before or on admission to the health care facility.

Documentation — The written record of nursing care including patient assessment; the actions taken as a result of that assessment; the plan of care developed and implemented; and the results of those actions. Documentation serves as the main, retrievable communication tool for the health care team.

Do-not-resuscitate (DNR) — A form of advance directives that outlines a patient's wishes for end-of-life decisions. "Allow natural death" (AND) better represents the patient's decision not to have "heroic measures" implemented to prolong life, and may be used in place of DNR.

Evidence-based practice (EBP) — Practices with outcomes that have been validated by research.

Family — For the purposes of this guide, "family" includes significant others and extended family.

Hand-off — The transfer of information (along with authority and responsibility) during transitions in care across the continuum for the purpose of ensuring the continuity and safety of the patient's care.

Health care team — The providers of patient care services who are required to provide direct patient care to help the patient achieve a positive outcome. Support services include, but are not limited to, pharmacy, radiology, blood bank, housekeeping, etc.

Health Insurance Portability and Accountability Act of 1996 (HIPAA) — Provides federal protection for personal health information, whether electronic, written, or oral. Disclosure of personal health information needed for patient care and other important purposes is permitted.

I PASS the BATON — A standardized method of organizing thoughts and communication using the following components: **I**nformation, **P**atient **A**ssessment, **S**ituation, **S**afety concerns, **B**ackground, **A**ction, **T**iming, **O**wnership, **N**ext.

The Joint Commission (TJC) — The independent accrediting organization that designates acceptable patient care and evaluates health care facilities' abilities to adhere to specific guidelines (e.g., documentation, processes, policies, and procedures). (www. jointcommission.org)

Knowledge — Defined as an organized body of information, usually of a factual or procedural nature, which, if applied, makes adequate performance of a job possible. Possession of knowledge does not ensure its proper application.

MAPS — A standardized method for organizing patient data: **M**edications, **A**llergies, **P**rocedure/**P**ertinent information, **S**pecial needs.

National Patient Safety Goals (NPSG) — Established by The Joint Commission to stimulate health care organizations' improvement processes addressing the most challenging patient safety issues.

"Never" events — Inexcusable adverse outcomes in a health care setting.

Patient Self-Determination Act (PSDA) — Requires Medicare and Medicaid providers to give adult individuals, at the time of inpatient admission or enrollment, certain information about their rights under state laws governing advance directives.

Perioperative Nursing Data Set (PNDS) — Standardized nursing vocabulary that addresses the perioperative patient experience from pre-admission until discharge.

Protected health information (HIPAA PHI) — Any information about health status, provision of health care, or payment for health care that can be linked to a specific individual, including any part of a patient's medical record or payment history. (www.hhs.gov/ocr/privacy/hipaa/understanding/summary/index.html)

Read back — A method to decrease errors resulting from verbal communication, including verbal and telephone orders and critical lab values. The information is written down by the receiver, and is then "read back" to the sender to confirm accuracy of the message.

Root cause analysis (RCA) — Problem-solving methods aimed at identifying the root causes of problems or events. The practice of RCA is predicated on the belief that problems are best solved by attempting to correct or eliminate root causes, as opposed to merely addressing the immediately obvious symptoms.

SBAR — A standardized communication process that includes **S**ituation, **B**ackground, **A**ssessment, and **R**ecommendations. It is especially useful when there is a need to prioritize actions related to recommendations for care.

SHARED — A method of organizing thought and communication through **S**ituation, **H**istory, **A**ssessment, **R**equest, **E**valuate, **D**ocument.

Standardized communication plan — An organized method of receiving and transmitting information, usually involving a checklist and an easily remembered acronym.

Surgical Care Improvement Project (SCIP) — A CDC/CMS multi-year national campaign with the goal of substantially reducing surgical morbidity and mortality through collaborative efforts.

SURPASS — A standardized, comprehensive communication tool: **SUR**gical **PA**tient **S**afety **S**ystem.

Universal Protocol — A procedure created by The Joint Commission to prevent wrong person, wrong procedure, wrong site surgery in hospitals and outpatient settings. The Universal Protocol consists of three steps:
1. A preoperative/preprocedure verification process
2. Marking the operative/procedure site
3. A time-out (final verification), which is performed immediately before starting the operation/procedure

WHO checklist — A surgical checklist containing items to be reviewed during crucial stages of the perioperative experience. The goal is to improve patient safety by adhering to proven standards of care.

References

American Nurses Association (ANA). (2004). *Nursing Scope and Standards of Practice.* Silver Spring, MD: ANA.

AORN. (2011). *Perioperative Nursing Data Set* (3rd ed.). Denver: AORN, Inc.

AORN. (2011). Position statement: Creating a practice environment of safety. Retrieved Feb. 21, 2014, from http://www.aorn.org/Clinical_Practice/Position_Statements/Position_Statements.aspx

AORN. (2014). Recommended practices for transfer of patient care information. In *Perioperative Standards and Recommended Practices*. Denver: AORN, Inc.

Institute for Healthcare Improvement. (2014, Feb 1). SBAR technique for communication: A situational briefing model. Retrieved Feb. 7, 2014, from http://www.ihi.org/resources/Pages/Tools/SBARTechniqueforCommunicationASituationalBriefingModel.aspx

Johnson, F., Logsdon, P., Fournier, K., et al. (2013). SWITCH for safety: Perioperative hand-off tools. *AORN Journal, 98*(5), 495-504.

 The Joint Commission. (2013). *Improving America's Hospitals: The Joint Commission's Annual Report on Quality and Safety*. Retrieved Feb. 21, 2014, from http://www. jointcommission.org/annualreport.aspx

The Joint Commission. (2009). *The Joint Commission Guide to Improving Staff Communication*. Oakbrook Terrace, IL: Joint Commission Resources.

NANDA International, Inc. Retrieved Feb. 21, 2014, from http://www.nanda.org

Phillips, N. (2013). *Berry and Kohn's Operating Room Technique* (12th ed.). St. Louis: Mosby.

Rothrock, J.C. (Ed.). (2015). *Alexander's Care of the Patient in Surgery* (15th ed.). St. Louis: Mosby.

Answers to Chapter 4 Activities

Module I: Verbal and nonverbal communication — Pages 143-147

Activity — Short Answer

For each closed-ended (directive) preoperative interview question, provide an associated open-ended (non-directive) question. Compare the differences in quality and quantity of information received utilizing both approaches.

Sample responses:
1. *When was the last time you had anything to eat or drink?*
2. *Tell me what your name is.*
3. *In your own words, tell me what type of surgery you're having.*
4. *What else can I help you with?*

  Source: Phillips, N. (2013). *Berry and Kohn's Operating Room Technique* (12th ed., pp. 374-378). St. Louis: Mosby.

Case Study Activity

1. What parts of Mr. J.'s assessment requires an immediate intervention?

Elevated WBCs; low-normal hemoglobin/hematocrit.

2. Use the SBAR (Situation, Background, Assessment, Recommendation) format to describe how you would communicate this information to the surgeon and anesthesia care provider.

Sample response, elevated WBCs:
S = Your patient, Mr. J., scheduled for a left total knee arthroplasty, has an elevated WBC count of 11.3 mm³ and a temp of 100° F.
B = He recently had a full-mouth dental extraction in preparation for dentures.
A = I am concerned that Mr. J. may have an infection that could affect the outcome of his surgery.
R = I'd like you to come assess him and review the plan of care.

Sample response, low-normal hemoglobin and hematocrit:
S = Your patient, Mr. J., has low-normal hemoglobin and hematocrit levels.
B = He is scheduled for a left total knee arthroplasty.
A = His hemoglobin is 14.4 g/dL and his hematocrit is 42.7%. Although his platelet count is normal, I am concerned about blood loss and its effect on his H&H.
R = Would you like to order a type and screen to save time in case we need to give blood?

Source: Rothrock, J.C. (Ed.). *Alexander's Care of the Patient in Surgery* (2015, 15th ed., pp. 28-29). St. Louis: Mosby.

Activity — Critical Thinking

1. Highlight the areas in the scenario in which breaks in communication or protocol influenced patient outcomes.

- *Operative side and site were marked in the preoperative area by the preoperative nurse.*
- *The patient was positioned, prepped, and draped without the surgeon present in the room.*
- *The nurse did not question the request to move the pedals to the other side of the bed.*
- *The nurse was out of the room during the time-out.*
- *The nurse documented the time-out had occurred, even though she was not in the room.*
- *The surgeon reviewed the consent, x-rays, and H&P after the procedure to discover that he had operated on the wrong side.*

2. For each highlighted area, provide an example of "speaking up" that may have helped avert the occurrence.

- *"The Joint Commission recommends that the person performing the procedure should mark the site. Let's have the doctor come back to confirm the correct site and side before I take the patient back."*
- *"Let's have the time-out when the surgeon is here to confirm the correct patient, side, and site."*
- *"I've placed the pedals based on a left-sided laminectomy. Is there a discrepancy concerning the correct surgical side?"*
- *"I'm going to wait to get those sutures until after the time-out. Everybody needs to be in the room and focused on our patient's surgery."*
- *"I can't document this time-out unless I am participating. Let's make sure everyone is ready."*

- ***"Let's review the consent, x-rays, and H&P as part of the time-out to make sure we have the correct patient, operation, and side."***

3. What should be done to prevent the above situation from reoccurring in the future?

- ***Provide education to all members of the surgical team on the importance of active involvement and open communication.***
- ***Perform a root cause analysis (RCA) to reveal the variables that contributed to this wrong-side surgery, including failed communication.***
- ***Based on the results of the RCA, revise the facility policy for wrong patient, wrong procedure, and wrong side surgery. Communicate the changes to the perioperative team.***
- ***Perform regular audits to evaluate compliance with policy.***
- ***Implement components of a just culture which encourage active communication between all members of the health care team, regardless of role.***

Source: Rothrock, J.C. (Ed.). *Alexander's Care of the Patient in Surgery* (2015, 15th ed., p. 19). St. Louis: Mosby.

Activity — Critical Thinking

As she leaves the room to get additional suture, the circulating nurse asks the student she is precepting to put sterile saline in the basin opened on the ring stand. When she returns, she sees an unopened bottle of sterile saline sitting in the basin. How could this break in technique have been avoided?

- ***Provide clearer instructions, such as, "Pour the sterile saline into the sterile basin, standing far enough away from the basin to avoid contaminating the field. Do not allow the saline to splash out of the basin."***
- ***The circulator should not have delegated this task to the student without first evaluating her competence in transferring liquids to the sterile field.***

Source: Rothrock, J.C. (Ed.). *Alexander's Care of the Patient in Surgery* (2015, 15th ed., p. 8). St. Louis: Mosby.

Module 2: Written communication — Pages 148-151

Activity — Search and Circle

Please circle the items on the schedule board that violate HIPAA regulations.

See the following page for answers

Time	Room	Patient	Dr.	Procedure/ Anesth
0730–0900	OR1	J. Brown (SS# 100-98-0004)	Smith	Laparoscopic cholecystectomy /General
0915–1145	OR1	J. Brown (SS# 999-00-1234)	Smith	Right carotid endarterectomy/General
1200–1330	OR1	Carl Johnson (Patient is HIV +)	Smith	Right inguinal hernia repair/Moderate Sedation
0730–0815	OR2	T. Adams (Call his mom at 719-800-1623 when he's in PACU)	Brats	Tonsillectomy/General
0730–0900	OR3	Shirley Nickle (e-mail postoperative instructions to smick@yahoo.org)	Short	Abdominal hysterectomy /General
0915–1045	OR#3	Carol D. (DOB 07/08/56)	Short	Abdominal hysterectomy /General

Source: U.S. Dept of Health and Human Services. (2003, May). Summary of the HIPAA Privacy Rule. Retrieved Feb. 21, 2014, from http://www.hhs.gov/ocr/privacy/hipaa/understanding/summary/

Activity — Critical Thinking

A patient is scheduled for an exploratory laparotomy for a possible perforated viscus. When you arrive to interview the patient, you find the patient confused about the scheduled surgical procedure and he asks to speak to the surgeon. The permit has been signed, but the surgeon is not immediately available. What is the most appropriate course of action?

The patient should not be transported to the OR until the surgeon has answered questions to the patient's satisfaction.

Source: Phillips, N. (2013). *Berry and Kohn's Operating Room Technique* (12th ed., pp. 45-47). St. Louis: Mosby.

Case Study Activity

You document in Mr. J.'s electronic medical record that an incident report (occurrence report) has been completed related to an incorrect suture count. From a legal standpoint, what are the ramifications of this documentation?

The contents of a patient's medical record are discoverable in a court of law. Incident or occurrence reports are considered part of the overall institution/department quality improvement initiative and constitute privileged, private information. The fact that an incident report was filled out should not be documented in the patient's permanent record.

Source: Phillips, N. (2013). *Berry and Kohn's Operating Room Technique* (12th ed., p. 50). St. Louis: Mosby.

CHAPTER 5:
Transfer of Care

> **Test Specifications:**
> **5% of CNOR test questions are based on Transfer of Care.**

Introduction

Patient transfer, also called patient hand-off, involves passing care of the patient from one health care professional to another. Transfers occur many times during a patient's stay, regardless of the type of facility or setting. The goal of patient transfer is seamless continuity of care — a hallmark of patient safety. The increase in same day surgery, shorter hospital stays, and an older and higher acuity patient population increase the potential for errors related to transfer.

This chapter will help you develop a plan that actively involves staff members, patients, and their families in the transfer process. Implementing an interdisciplinary approach to every phase of patient care is emphasized. The importance of postoperative patient education is stressed.

Module 1: Transfer of Care Among Team Members

Though it may seem a simple task to hand over responsibility for a patient from one caregiver to another, patient transfer is a complex process. When an omission in vital information occurs, it may contribute to an adverse outcome. A standardized and clearly defined method of relaying pertinent patient information among caregivers may decrease the incidence of miscommunication by providing timely, accurate information about a patient's care plan, treatment, current condition, and any recent or anticipated changes. The hand-off should involve a face-to-face exchange between caregivers and an opportunity to ask questions or verify information.

Competency Outcomes

To successfully complete the activities in this module, you will need to be able to:

1. Identify the components of transfer of patient care during the perioperative period.
2. Use a standardized reporting process for communicating pertinent patient information to the next health care provider.

Recommended Reading

Alexander's Care of the Patient in Surgery. (2015, 15th ed.), Chapter 2: Patient safety and risk management; Unit II: Surgical interventions.

Berry and Kohn's Operating Room Technique. (2013, 12th ed.), Chapter 11: Ambulatory surgery centers and alternative surgical locations; Chapter 25: Coordinated roles of the scrub person and the circulating nurse; Chapter 30: Postoperative patient care.

Perioperative Standards and Recommended Practices. (2014), Recommended practices: Transfer of patient care information.

Key Words

Communication, continuity of care, hand-off, interdisciplinary, transfer of care

Activity — Multiple Choice

For each of the following components related to transfer of care, identify in which phase of care this information should be provided. Some answers will be used more than once.

1. Verification of correct patient, site, and procedure ____

2. Surgical count status ____

A = Preoperative

3. Allergies
(e.g., medications, chemicals, foods, natural rubber latex) ____

B = Intraoperative

C = Postoperative

4. Special precautions (e.g., transmission-based precautions, positioning) ____

5. Presence or absence of complications associated with this surgery ____

6. Specimens ____

7. Communication with family or significant other(s) ____

8. Required legal and clinical documentation (e.g., history & physical, informed consent) ____

9. Performance measures (e.g., prophylactic antibiotics, DVT prophylaxis) ____

10. Thermal interventions ____

Case Study Activity

Complete the hand-off form on the following two pages as part of your transfer of care for Mr. J.

PATIENT HAND-OFF FORM
Memorial Hospital

Name: _____ Age: _____ Surgeon: _____

Preoperative RN to Intraoperative RN Hand-Off Tool

Planned surgical procedure: _____ **Code status:** _____

Surgical procedure verified/marked: Site: _____ Side: _____

Planned anesthesia type:

☐ Local ☐ Peripheral ☐ MAC ☐ Regional ☐ General

Required documents present:

☐ Consent ☐ H&P ☐ Labs ☐ Advanced directive ☐ X-rays

Abnormal tests/labs: _____

☐ Surgeon notified ☐ Anesthesia care provider notified

Allergies: ☐ Yes _____ ☐ NKDA

Home medications: _____

Significant medical history: _____

Previous surgeries (type and date): _____

Any complications? ☐ N/A Type and date: _____

VS: BP____ R____ T____ P____ O$_2$ sat____ Pain____

Mental status:

☐ Alert, oriented X3 ☐ Other (describe) _____

Sensory deficit:

☐ None ☐ Hearing ☐ Visual ☐ Tactile ☐ Verbal

Special needs:

☐ Communication _____

☐ Cultural _____

☐ Spiritual/Religious _____

Musculoskeletal/skin assessment:

☐ Intact

☐ Describe any impairments to integrity: _____

Fall risk: ☐ Yes ☐ No

IV: Fluid _____ Site _____

Meds given preop:

☐ N/A ☐ Other: _____

Blood products available:

☐ N/A ☐ Type and screen ☐ Type and cross ☐ Whole blood units _____

☐ Packed cells units _____ ☐ Other: _____

SCIP initiatives:

☐ DVT prophylaxis ☐ Beta blocker ☐ BS monitoring

☐ Antibiotic: Type _____ Time _____

Family/significant other name(s): _____

☐ Surgeon spoke with ☐ In waiting room

☐ Contact information _____

Report given to _____ **RN by** _____ **RN**

Intraoperative RN to Postanesthesia Care RN Hand-Off Tool

Procedure: _____ **Surgeon:** _____

Code status: _____

Allergies: ☐ Yes _____ ☐ NKDA

Significant medical history: _____

Previous surgeries (type and date): _____

Current meds: _____

Meds given intraop:

☐ Antibiotic: Type _____ Time: _____

☐ Pain: Type _____ Time: _____

☐ Other: Type _____ Time: _____

IV: Fluid_____ Site _____

Blood given:

☐ N/A ☐ Whole blood units _____ Time: _____

☐ Packed cells units _____ Time: _____

Other:_____ Time: _____

Drain/catheter/tubing: Site_____ Type_____

Assessment of skin integrity: (include pressure points, positioning related areas, and incision site)

☐ Skin intact

☐ Other:_____ Surgeon notified _____

☐ Dressing/cast/splint: Type_____ Site _____

Restrictions:

☐ Yes Type: _____

☐ NA

Pain management plan:

☐ PCA

☐ IV

☐ Regional block

☐ Peripheral nerve block

Anticipated labs/tests/treatments: _____

Issues/concerns: _____

Family name(s):_____

☐ In waiting room

☐ Contact information _____

Report given to _____ **RN by** _____ **RN**

"Go To" Activity — Skill Building

Review how your facility updates families on a family member's progress in the OR/procedural area.

Represent your perioperative department by participating in postoperative patient rounds.

Compare your facility's current practice on communicating patient care information with AORN's recommended practices for transfer of patient care information.

Additional Readings/Resources

AMA. (2014). Resources on improving patient hand offs. Retrieved Feb. 20, 2014, from http://www.ama-assn.org/ama/pub/about-ama/our-people/member-groups-sections/resident-fellow-section/rfs-resources/patient-handoffs.page
Note: Includes articles, videos, and resources for improving patient care.

AORN. (2013). Patient Hand Off Tool Kit. Retrieved Feb. 20, 2014, from http://www.aorn.org/PracticeResources/ToolKits/PatientHandOffToolKit/

Criscitelli, T. (2013). Safe patient hand-off strategies. *AORN Journal, 97(5)*, 582-585.

Johnson, F., Logsdon, P., Fournier, K., et al. (2013). SWITCH for safety: Perioperative hand-off tools. *AORN Journal, 98(5)*, 494-507.

Micheli, A.J., Curran-Campbell, S., & Connor, L. (2010). The evolution of a surgical liaison program in a children's hospital. *AORN Journal, 92(2)*, 158-168.

Seifert, P.C. (2012). Implementing AORN recommended practices for transfer of patient care information. *AORN Journal, 96(5)*, 475-493.

Stefan, K.A. (2010). The nurse liaison in perioperative services: A family-centered approach. *AORN Journal, 92(2)*, 150-157.

Module 2: Discharge Planning for the Patient Leaving the Facility

Every patient and family is entitled to discharge planning services that are appropriate and individualized to their needs. Federal and state requirements often affect specific components of the individualized discharge plan. The discharge plan should address:

- any aftercare services needed, including the need for supervision after discharge and any support services needed;
- information about the medications prescribed and how to use them appropriately; and
- the plan for any follow-up care that is needed.

In addition to rights, patients also have a responsibility to participate as fully as possible in the discharge planning process. The perioperative nurse should assess patient/caregiver needs, individualize the postoperative plan of care, and encourage the patient and caregivers to participate whenever feasible.

Competency Outcomes

To successfully complete the activities in this module, you will need to be able to:

1. Incorporate recommended standards and regulatory requirements into discharge planning.
2. Provide patient and family postoperative education based on assessed needs.

Recommended Reading

Alexander's Care of the Patient in Surgery. (2015, 15th ed.), Chapter 10: Postoperative patient care and pain management; Chapter 26: Pediatric surgery; Chapter 27: Geriatric surgery.

Berry and Kohn's Operating Room Technique. (2013, 12th ed.), Chapter 11: Ambulatory surgery centers and alternative surgical locations; Chapter 30: Perianesthesia and post-procedural patient care.

Key Words

Collaboration, discharge planning, education, health literacy, interdisciplinary, pain management, postoperative plan of care, regulatory guidelines, wound care

Activity — Critical Thinking

1. You are employed in an office-based surgery setting. What general discharge instructions should be provided for a healthy 26-year-old woman who has just had a small lipoma removed from her left forearm?

2. How would your answer to question #1 above differ if your patient was a 5-year-old girl who had just had debridement and repair of laceration left knee from a bicycle accident?

Case Study Activity

1. Mr. J. is hard of hearing. How can you assist him in understanding his discharge instructions?

2. Based on Mr. J.'s increased risk for development of a DVT, what instructions should he receive prior to discharge?

Activity — Critical Thinking

PZ, a 55-year-old woman, is scheduled to undergo repair of a torn left rotator cuff as an ambulatory procedure. She is the sole caretaker for her frail, elderly mother who lives with her. PZ states that it is important to both of them that her mother remains at home.

PZ is 5 feet tall and weighs 165 pounds. She smokes one pack of cigarettes per day and was diagnosed a year ago with obstructive sleep apnea (OSA). PZ reports that she has difficulty wearing the continuous positive airway pressure (CPAP) mask that she was given when her OSA was diagnosed. She also has elevated blood pressure, but it is managed with medication. She reports that she can become sleepy during the day and often must take naps.

PZ injured her shoulder assisting her mother with routine activities of daily living (ADLs) and delayed seeing a surgeon because of her caretaker responsibilities. As a consequence, she is quite uncomfortable and rates the level of her pain as an 8 on a scale of 0 to 10. She is looking forward to having the repair done so that she can regain lost function and reduce or eliminate her shoulder pain. However, she worries about how her recovery will affect her ability to care for her mother.

1. When should discharge planning begin?

2. How does PZ's diagnosis of OSA influence the planned procedure?

3. What immediate goals should be addressed in the discharge plan of care, and how can they be approached in an interdisciplinary manner with PZ?

4. What are the educational needs associated with PZ's postoperative plan of care, and how should this information be presented?

"Go To" Activity — Skill Building

Volunteer to talk with patients and their families about their surgical experiences during hospital tours or preoperative visits.

Assist with follow-up phone calls to discharged patients. What are the most frequent questions, concerns, and complications voiced by your patients? How can this information be incorporated to improve care for future patients?

Talk with a case manager or social worker about his or her job. Incorporate discharge planning into the perioperative plan of care by anticipating and addressing potential problems with the appropriate discipline.

Additional Readings/Resources

Flanagan, J. (2009). Postoperative telephone calls: Timing is everything. *AORN Journal, 90*(1), 41-51.

Girard, N.J. (2013). Discharge instructions in the PACU: Who remembers? *AORN Journal, 98*(5), 554, 448.

The Joint Commission. (2010). *Advancing Effective Communication, Cultural Competence, and Patient- and Family-Centered Care: A Roadmap for Hospitals.* Oakbrook Terrace, IL: The Joint Commission. Retrieved Feb. 20, 2014, from http://www.jointcommission.org/assets/1/6/ARoadmap forHospitalsfinalversion727.pdf

The Joint Commission. (2012, June). *Hot Topics in Health Care, Transitions of Care: The need for a more effective approach to continuing patient care.* Retrieved Feb. 20, 2014, from http://www.jointcommission.org/assets/1/18/Hot_Topics_Transitions_of_Care.pdf

Monachos, C.L. (2007). Assessing and addressing low health literacy among surgical outpatients. *AORN Journal, 90*(2), 373-383.

Nelson, J.M., & Carrington, J.M. (2011). Transitioning the older adult in the ambulatory care setting. *AORN Journal, 94*(4), 348-361.

Rouse, C.L., & Bardelman, K. (2009). Collaborative care planning. *AORN Journal, 89*(6), 1115-1120.

Talsma, A., Anderson, C., Geun, H., et al. (2013). Evaluation of OR staffing and postoperative patient outcomes. *AORN Journal, 97*(2), 230-242.

Taylor, E. (2008). Providing developmentally based care for toddlers. *AORN Journal, 87*(5), 992-999.

Taylor, E. (2009). Providing developmentally based care for preschoolers. *AORN Journal, 88*(2), 267-273.

Taylor, E. (2009). Providing developmentally based care for school-aged and adolescent patients. *AORN Journal, 90*(2), 261-267.

Vealey-Amato, E.J., Fountain, P., & Coppola, D. (2012). Perfecting patient flow in the surgical setting. *AORN Journal, 96*(1), 46-57.

Chapter Summary

Effective discharge planning for the patient undergoing an operative or invasive procedure is an evolving process, starting when the patient initially agrees to undergo the procedure and ending when recovery is complete. A well-planned, thorough, standardized transfer process based on patient needs is more consistently implemented regardless of setting.

The perioperative nurse contributes to the discharge plan of care by identifying appropriate desired outcomes related to the patient and the procedure, and by actively collaborating with other members of the health care team to help the patient and family achieve those outcomes as fully as possible. Appropriate and effective discharge planning is a key component of returning the patient to an optimal level of wellness.

Glossary

Ambulatory surgery — For purposes of this guide, "ambulatory surgery" includes outpatient surgery, same-day surgery, day surgery, etc.

Discharge planning — The process of assessing the needs of patients for post-procedure care, developing a coordinated and multidisciplinary plan to provide the care required (including patient and family education, available services, and referral agencies and support groups), and evaluating the plan. The process begins before or on admission to the health care facility.

Documentation — The written record (e.g., paper or electronic) of nursing care including patient assessment, the actions taken as a result of that assessment, the plan of care developed and implemented, and the results of those actions. Documentation serves as the main, retrievable communication tool for the health care team.

Family — For purposes of this guide, "family" includes significant others and extended family.

Health literacy — The ability to apply information in making health care decisions.

Interdisciplinary collaboration — A process of joint decision making and communication among health care providers with the mutual goal of satisfying the needs of the patient while respecting the unique abilities of each person involved in the care. Trust, knowledge, mutual respect, cooperation, coordination, shared responsibility, good communication skills, and optimism are desired traits of the multidisciplinary team.

National Patient Safety Goals — Established initially in 2002 and now updated annually by The Joint Commission in an effort to assist health care facilities in addressing specific areas of concern related to identified patient safety issues.

Outcome criteria — Statements developed to identify the tasks or conditions to be implemented that will assist the patient in achieving the desired outcomes. Outcome criteria indicate an expected, measurable change in the patient's health status.

Perioperative Nursing Data Set: The Perioperative Nursing Vocabulary (PNDS) — A guidebook that provides nursing diagnoses, nursing interventions, and patient outcomes statements specific to the perioperative environment.

References

AORN. (2011). *Perioperative Nursing Data Set* (3rd ed.). Denver: AORN, Inc.

AORN. (2014). *Perioperative Standards and Recommended Practices*. Denver: AORN, Inc.

Phillips, N. (2013). *Berry and Kohn's Operating Room Technique*. (12th ed.). St. Louis: Mosby.

Rothrock, J.C. (Ed.). (2015). *Alexander's Care of the Patient in Surgery* (15th ed.). St. Louis: Mosby.

Answers to Chapter 5 Activities

Module 1: Transfer of care between team members — Pages 159-163

Activity — Multiple Choice

For each of the following components related to transfer of care, identify in which phase of care this information should be provided. Some answers will be used more than once.

A = preoperative   B = intraoperative   C = postoperative

1. Verification of correct patient, site, and procedure: ***A, B, C***

2. Surgical count status: ***B***

3. Allergies (e.g., medications, chemicals, foods, natural rubber latex): ***A, B, C***

4. Special precautions (e.g., transmission-based precautions, positioning): ***A, B, C***

5. Presence or absence of complications associated with this surgery: ***C***

6. Specimens: ***B***

7. Communication with family or significant other(s): ***A, B, C***

8. Required legal and clinical documentation (e.g., history and physical, informed consent): ***A***

9. Performance measures (e.g., prophylactic antibiotics, DVT prophylaxis): ***A, B, C***

10. Thermal interventions: ***A, B, C***

> Source: AORN. (2014). Recommended practices for transfer of patient care information. In *Perioperative Standards and Recommended Practices*, pp. 502-503. Denver: AORN, Inc.

Module 2: Discharge planning for the patient leaving the facility — Pages 164-168

Activity — Critical Thinking

1. You are employed in an office-based surgery setting. What general discharge instructions should be provided for a healthy 26-year-old woman who has just had a small lipoma removed from her left forearm?

Pain control methods, both pharmacologic and non-pharmacologic; side effects of any medications ordered; wound and dressing care; activity level; signs and symptoms of infection; when and whom to contact for additional assistance/questions/concerns; when to return to doctor's office or clinic for suture removal; any other information based on specific patient needs.

Source: Rothrock, J.C. (Ed.). (2015). *Alexander's Care of the Patient in Surgery* (15th ed., p. 293). St. Louis: Mosby.

2. How would your answer to question #1 above differ if your patient was a 5-year-old girl who had just had debridement and repair of laceration left knee from a bicycle accident?

The parents or guardians will be included in postoperative teaching. Activity restrictions include when the child could return to school or day care and any limitations on running or physical contact while playing. Demonstrate wound care on a stuffed animal or doll. Allow the child to handle any objects that will be used in care (e.g., temporal or tympanic membrane thermometer). Identify the method the child will use to communicate pain (words like "ouch" or "owie") and/or the use of a pain scale such as FACES. Put a similar dressing or band-aid on the child's personal stuffed animal or toy. Encourage fluids and easy-to-digest foods. The child may exhibit increased separation anxiety or regression immediately after the procedure and require additional comfort measures from caregivers. Use popular cartoon, movie, or storybook characters and terminology to help describe experiences and reinforce postoperative teaching.

Sources: Rothrock, J.C. (Ed.). (2015). *Alexander's Care of the Patient in Surgery* (15th ed., pp.1008-1018). St. Louis: Mosby; Phillips, N. (2013). *Berry and Kohn's Operating Room Technique,* pp. 127-135, 159. St. Louis: Mosby.

Case Study Activity

1. Mr. J. is hard of hearing. How can you assist him in understanding his discharge instructions?

Ensure that Mr. J.'s hearing aids are in place and functioning. Face Mr. J. when speaking to him and speak slowly and clearly. Make sure Mr. J. is comfortable and that the environment is quiet and conducive to learning. Use visual teaching aids (pamphlets with large type, videos, manipulatives) to augment verbal instructions. Plan teaching sessions when a family member is present. Utilize the "teach-back" method to determine Mr. J.'s understanding of his postoperative care.

Source: Rothrock, J.C. (Ed.). (2015). *Alexander's Care of the Patient in Surgery* (15th ed., pp. 1098-1099). St. Louis: Mosby.

2. Based on Mr. J.'s increased risk for development of a DVT, what instructions should he receive prior to discharge?

1. Identification of signs and symptoms of DVT (e.g., leg pain, swelling, unexplained shortness of breath, wheezing, chest pain, palpitations, anxiety, sweating, or coughing up blood)
2. Emergency health care provider contact information
3. Appropriate administration of anticoagulant medication (this may include teaching Mr. J. how to give himself an injection)
4. Stress the importance of early ambulation and passive and active range of motion of lower extremities.
5. Avoiding clothing or activities that restrict circulation of lower extremities
6. Schedule any follow-up lab work

Source: AORN. (2014). Recommended practices for prevention of deep vein thrombosis. In *Perioperative Standards and Recommended Practices*, p. 426. Denver: AORN, Inc.

Activity — Critical Thinking

PZ, a 55-year-old woman, is scheduled to undergo repair of a torn left rotator cuff as an ambulatory procedure. She is the sole caretaker for her frail, elderly mother who lives with her. PZ states that it is important to both of them that her mother remains at home.

PZ is 5 feet tall and weighs 165 pounds. She smokes one pack of cigarettes per day and was diagnosed a year ago with obstructive sleep apnea (OSA). PZ reports that she has difficulty wearing the continuous positive airway pressure (CPAP) mask that she was given when her OSA was diagnosed. She also has elevated blood pressure, but it is managed with medication. She reports that she can become sleepy during the day and often must take naps.

PZ injured her shoulder assisting her mother with routine activities of daily living (ADLs) and delayed seeing a surgeon because of her caretaker responsibilities. As a consequence, she is quite uncomfortable and rates the level of her pain as an 8 on a scale of 0 to 10. She is looking forward to having the repair done so that she can regain lost function and reduce or eliminate her shoulder pain. However, she worries about how her recovery will affect her ability to care for her mother.

1. When should discharge planning begin?

Discharge planning for PZ should begin in the surgeon's office when she agrees to have her rotator cuff repaired.

2. How does PZ's diagnosis of OSA influence the planned procedure?

PZ's OSA diagnosis is significant because it may affect her ability to have the procedure done on an ambulatory basis, and it will influence the type of anesthesia selected. She should plan on being monitored in the hospital overnight to prevent poor outcomes. The surgeon's office staff may need to work with PZ's insurer to obtain precertification for admission to avoid possible cancellation of her procedure.

3. What immediate goals should be addressed in the discharge plan of care, and how can they be approached in an interdisciplinary manner with PZ?

PZ's immediate goals for discharge planning would include:
1. Pain management and control to an acceptable level
2. Prevention of postoperative infection
3. Address mother's needs in terms of home care or short-term stay in assisted living facility
4. Maintenance of current home meds to control hypertension
5. Re-evaluation of CPAP mask fit
6. Follow-up appointment with surgeon
7. Contact information of person to call in case of emergency/questions related to postoperative care

Secondary goals include:
Return to optimal function

Weight loss and smoking cessation counseling
Respite care as needed for mother

These goals are addressed by a variety of caregivers, including physicians, nutritionists, social workers, and nurses.

4. What are the educational needs associated with PZ's postoperative plan of care, and how should this information be presented?

The educational needs associated with PZ's situation are primarily focused on pain management, wound healing, and regaining function. Pharmacologic and nonpharmacologic approaches to managing pain and realistic expectations for long-term pain control should be reviewed in terms that PZ can easily understand. Providing information in a variety of formats (verbal, written, video, etc.) will aid in retention of material. Signs and symptoms of wound infection should be reviewed, along with information on how smoking negatively affects wound healing and increases the risk for infection. Part of the recovery process for PZ will be regaining function in her shoulder, so she must clearly understand any prescribed postoperative exercises and set up an appointment for physical therapy after the procedure.

NOTES

CHAPTER 6:
Cleaning, Disinfecting, Packaging, Sterilizing, Transporting, and Storing Instruments and Supplies

Test Specifications:
12% of CNOR test questions are based on Cleaning, Disinfecting, Packaging, Sterilizing, Transporting, and Storing Instruments and Supplies.

Introduction

The defining characteristic of the perioperative arena is its sterile environment that protects patients during surgical procedures. The perioperative nurse has the unique responsibility to create a sterile field and ensure its continued sterility until the patient's skin integrity is restored and he/she is safe from harm from exposure to pathogens. Appropriate sterilization and disinfection of instruments and equipment in that sterile field protect both patients and perioperative personnel from exposure to infectious material.

Disinfection and sterilization is an area where the professional perioperative nurse understands the interactive nature of a multidisciplinary environment and how one discipline can influence the effectiveness of another. Although the disinfection and sterilization of instruments is usually done in a sterile processing department (SPD), perioperative nurses participate actively in ensuring that the instruments and equipment are effectively processed. Processing of instruments and equipment begins at the point of use. Everyone who handles sterile instrumentation and equipment participates in the process.

The perioperative nurse who has knowledge of the principles and practices involved in infection prevention, and the legal and regulatory requirements that impact the practice, is well prepared to think critically and make effective practice decisions about cleaning, disinfecting, packaging, sterilizing, transporting, and storing instruments and supplies.

This chapter will challenge your critical thinking and decision-making skills related to current infection prevention and disinfection and sterilization practices. Applying these principles and practices will help you protect your patient and reduce the risk of surgical site infections. This chapter will also prepare you to ensure the sterility of instruments and equipment delivered to the sterile field regardless of where they were processed.

Module 1: Microbiological Considerations Related to Infection Control Principles

Introduction

Any microorganism can be pathogenic if it invades a susceptible area. The skin and mucous membranes are the body's primary protection against infection.

The most common source of pathogens found in surgical site infections is the patient's own flora (CDC, 1999); however, pathogens can be introduced onto the sterile field from other sources, including contaminated instruments, supplies, or other people. Proper sterilization and disinfection practices disrupt the chain of infection by removing pathogens.

Perioperative personnel also are at risk for exposure to pathogens. Personal protective equipment and good aseptic technique protect personnel from contamination and infection. Studies have demonstrated that double-gloving can reduce personnel exposure to pathogens via needlesticks (AORN, 2014, pp. 95-96).

In addition to the common infectious agents encountered in the OR, there are always new and challenging microorganisms. Microorganisms that have developed resistance to common antibiotics have evolved into pathogens such as methicillin-resistant *Staphylococcus aureus* (MRSA), vancomycin-resistant *Enterococcus* (VRE), carbapenem-resistant enterobacteriaceae (CRE), and multidrug-resistant *Mycobacterium tuberculosis* (MDR-TB) that require special attention. The prion responsible for transmissible spongiform encephalopathy (i.e., Creutzfeld-Jacob disease) is not destroyed using routine procedures for disinfection and sterilization of surgical instruments. We will continue to be challenged to protect our patients and ourselves as microorganisms adapt to our efforts to eradicate them.

Competency Outcomes

To successfully complete the activities in this module, you will need to be able to:

1. Choose appropriate personal protective equipment (PPE) required to reduce the risk of transmitting infectious organisms.
2. Describe the proper management of patients with known or suspected transmissible infections.

Recommended Readings

Alexander's Care of the Patient in Surgery. (2015, 15th ed.), Chapter 4: Infection prevention and control.

Berry and Kohn's Operating Room Technique. (2013, 12th ed.), Chapter 14: Surgical microbiology and antimicrobial therapy; Chapter 15: Principles of asepsis and sterile technique; Chapter 16: Appropriate attire, surgical hand hygiene, and gowning and gloving.

Perioperative Standards and Recommended Practices. (2014), Recommended practices:
- High level disinfection.
- Prevention of transmissible infections.

Key Words

Airborne precautions, antisepsis, carbapenem-resistant enterobacteriaceae (CRE), chain of infection, contact precautions, Creutzfeld-Jacob disease (CJD), droplet precautions, methicillin-resistant *Staphylococcus aureus* (MRSA), multidrug-resistant *Mycobacterium tuberculosis* (MDR-TB), pathogen, personal protective equipment (PPE), standard precautions, transmission-based precautions, vancomycin-resistant *Enterococcus* (VRE)

Activity — Fill in the Blank

What is considered the most important and effective intervention for preventing

infections? _____.

Activity — Stop the Spread! Part 1

For each of the following diseases, choose the appropriate transmission-based precautions.

Human immunodeficiency virus (HIV) _____   A. Contact

Mycobacterium tuberculosis _____   B. Droplet

Hepatitis B _____   A. Airborne

Staphylococcus aureus _____

Clostridium difficile _____

Pseudomonas _____

Varicella _____

Influenza _____

Activity — Stop the Spread! Part 2

Draw a line between each type of precaution and its appropriate method of preventing transmission. Use each answer only once.

Standard   Standard + mask

Contact   Hand hygiene; PPE if risk for exposure to blood/body fluids

Droplet   Standard + N95 respirator

Airborne   Standard + gloves, gown

Activity — Critical Thinking

You have just cared for a patient who is suspected of having Creutzfeld-Jacob disease (CJD). What is the preferred method for inactivating prions on semi-critical and critical devices exposed to high-infectivity tissue?

"Go To" Activity — Skill Building

Talk with the infection preventionist or the director of infection prevention in your facility about tracking and surveillance methods for infectious diseases and surgical site infections.

Volunteer to represent your department at your facility's infection prevention committee.

Review your department's policies and procedures on standard and transmission-based precautions. Compare them to CDC and AORN standards.

Case Study Activity

In evaluating Mr. J., what risk factors for a surgical site infection do you find?

"Go To" Activity — Check It Out!

Go to Question #16, Infection control; Question #23, Transmission-based precautions; Question #37, CJD; and Questions #48 and #49, Percutaneous injuries, Parts I and II, under the Perioperative question of the week tab in the Toolbox at http://www.cc-institute.org/toolbox for additional critical-thinking questions.

Additional Readings/Resources

Benson, S.M., Novak, D.A., & Ogg, M.J. (2013). Proper use of surgical N95 respirators and surgical masks in the OR. *AORN Journal, 97*(4), 457-470.

Centers for Disease Control and Prevention (CDC). Healthcare-associated infections. Retrieved Feb. 18, 2014, from http://www.cdc.gov/HAI/ssi/ssi.html
Note: Contains resources for preventing surgical site infections.

Durai, R., Ng, P.C.H., & Hoque, H. (2010). Methicillin-resistant *Staphylococcus aureus*: An update. *AORN Journal, 91*(5), 599-609.

Freeman, S.S., Lara, G.L., Courts, M.R., Wanzer, L.J., et al. (2009). An evidence-based process for evaluating infection control policies. *AORN Journal, 89*(3), 489-507.

Lassiter, S. (2011). Preventing infection: Collaboration between surgical team members and infection preventionists. *AORN Journal, 93*(2), 287-290.

Lipke, V.L., & Hyott, A.S. (2010). Reducing surgical site infections by bundling multiple risk reduction strategies and active surveillance. *AORN Journal, 92*(3), 288-296.

Murphy, R.J. (2012). Preventing multi-drug-resistant Gram-negative organisms in surgical patients. *AORN Journal, 96*(3), 315-329.

Siegel. J.D., Rhinehart E., Jackson, M., et al. and the Healthcare Infection Control Practices Advisory Committee. (2007). Guideline for Isolation Precautions: Preventing Transmission of Infectious Agents in Healthcare Settings. Retrieved Feb. 19, 2014, from http://www.cdc.gov/hicpac/pdf/isolation/Isolation2007.pdf

Stanton, C. (2010). Advancing infection prevention in the ambulatory setting. *AORN Journal, 92*(6), S73-S77.

Vasaly, F.W., & Reines, H.D. (2009). A quality committee's evaluation of surgical intervention for *Clostridium difficile* infection. *AORN Journal, 90*(2), 192-204.

Module 2: Cleaning and Disinfecting Instruments and Supplies

Introduction

The process of disinfection or sterilization starts with cleaning. An item can be clean without being sterile, but no item can be sterile without being clean. Similarly, you can clean without disinfecting, but cannot disinfect without cleaning. The risk for transmitting infection is taken into account when determining the level and type of disinfection.

Facilities often manage borrowed or consigned ("loaner") instruments. Vendors may provide instrumentation for a new procedure on a trial basis, or special instrumentation for a unique procedure. A comprehensive policy to manage loaner instruments ensures that they are received in sufficient time and are properly processed on site in the same manner as facility-owned instruments.

Competency Outcomes

To successfully complete the activities in this module, you will need to be able to:

1. Recognize the influence of professional and regulatory agencies in developing practice standards related to safe processing of surgical instruments and supplies.
2. Identify infection control principles related to the cleaning and disinfection of surgical instruments and supplies.

Recommended Readings

Alexander's Care of the Patient in Surgery. (2015, 15th ed.), Chapter 4: Infection prevention and control.

Berry and Kohn's Operating Room Technique. (2013, 12th ed.), Chapter 17: Decontamination and disinfection.

Perioperative Standards and Recommended Practices. (2014), Guidance statements:
• Environmental responsibility.
• Role of the health care industry representative.

Perioperative Standards and Recommended Practices. (2014), Recommended practices:
• Cleaning and processing flexible endoscopes.
• Cleaning and care of instruments and powered equipment.
• High level disinfection.
• Sterilization.

Key Words

AAMI, bioburden, cleaning, critical item, decontamination, disinfection, documentation, enzymatic cleaner, FDA, germicide, high-level disinfection, loaner instrumentation, low-level disinfection, non-critical item, semi-critical item, Spaulding classification

Activity — Multiple Choice

Circle the most reliable source for information regarding processing of instruments and equipment.

A. OSHA regulations

C. FDA protocols

B. TJC requirements

D. Manufacturers' instructions

Activity — Matching

Match the item to its definition.

1. Non-critical _____

2. Semi-critical _____

3. Critical _____

A. Enters sterile tissues including the vascular system

B. Contacts non-intact skin and mucous membranes

C. Contacts intact skin or does not come in contact with the patient

Activity — Put It In Its Place

Match the following items to the potential for transmitting infection and their appropriate method of processing.

Blood pressure cuff	Laparoscope	Tourniquet cuff
Laryngoscope	Doppler	Colonoscope
Balfour retractor	Mayo stand	

Disease transmission risk	Item(s)	Method of processing
Non-critical	_____	Intermediate-level disinfection
Semi-critical	_____	High-level disinfection
Critical	_____	Sterilization

Activity — Do You Know?

Check all of the following that represent proper management of instruments used during a surgical procedure.

_____A. Cleaning of instruments begins in the Sterile Processing Department (SPD).

_____B. Instruments containing multiple parts should be returned for cleaning and disinfection in one piece to minimize risk of displacing one of the parts.

_____C. Isolate and mark instruments in need of repair.

_____D. Opened but unused instruments do not need to be decontaminated.

_____E. Soak used items in enzymatic detergent or spray per manufacturer's recommendations to prevent drying of bioburden.

Activity — Scramble

Number the following steps in high-level disinfection in the correct order:

_____Flush lumens with the disinfectant.

_____Clean the instrument.

_____Time the immersion cycle.

_____Wear appropriate PPE.

_____Document results of processing.

_____Check solution for minimum effective concentration.

_____Deliver to point of use without contaminating.

_____Rinse with sterile water.

_____Immerse instrument in disinfectant according to manufacturer's recommendations.

Activity — Short Answer

How long can an item that has been high-level disinfected be stored before use?

Activity — Critical Thinking

A surgical instrumentation vendor arrives at 0715 for your scheduled 0730 anterior/posterior spinal fusion case with a set of implants. The implants have been sterilized at another facility and are covered with a heavy plastic dust cover. What is your response?

"Go To" Activity — Skill Building

Locate and review the Association for the Advancement of Medical Instrumentation (AAMI), *Comprehensive Guide to Steam Sterilization and Sterility Assurance in Health Care Facilities,* in your sterile processing, infection prevention, or biomed department.

Spend an afternoon in your sterile processing department. Compare cleaning, disinfection, packaging, and sterilization methods to those outlined in AORN's standards and recommended practices.

Review your policy on loaner instrumentation and compare it with AORN's standards and recommended practices. How is compliance with this policy tracked?

Review your immediate-use sterilization log for trends; recommend purchasing additional inventory for instruments that are routinely sterilized for immediate use.

"Go To" Activity — Check It Out!

Go to Question #21, Reprocessing opened and unused supplies; Question #33, Count sheets in trays; and Question #46, TASS, under the Perioperative question of the week tab in the Toolbox at http://www.cc-institute.org/toolbox for critical-thinking exercises.

Additional Readings/Resources

Allen, G. (Ed.). (2010). Infection prevention in the perioperative setting: Zero tolerance for infections. *Perioperative Nursing Clinics, 5*(4).

Azizi, J., Anderson, S.G., Murphy, S., et al. (2012). Uphill grime: Process improvement in surgical instrument cleaning. *AORN Journal, 98*(6), 152-162.

Burlingame, B. (2009). Reprocessing flexible endoscopes before use. *AORN Journal, 89*(2), 403-405.

Centers for Disease Control and Prevention (CDC). (2008). Healthcare Infection Practices Advisory Committee (HICPAC). Guideline for disinfection and sterilization in healthcare facilities. Retrieved Feb. 18, 2014, from http://www.cdc.gov/hicpac/Disinfection_Sterilization/toc.html

Cuming, R.G., Rocco, T.S., & McEachem, A.G. (2008). Improving compliance with Occupational Safety and Health Administration Standards. *AORN Journal, 87*(2), 347-360.

Denholm, B. (2009). Bypassing decontamination of the outer rigid instrument container. *AORN Journal, 90*(5), 755.

Goodman, T. (Ed.). (2010). Sterilization and disinfection for the perioperative nurse. *Perioperative Nursing Clinics, 5*(3).

IAHCSMM. Position paper on the management of loaner instrumentation. Retrieved Feb. 18, 2014, from http://www.iahcsmm.org/pdfs/IAHCSMM_Position_Paper_%20 Management_of_Loaner_Instrumentation_070111.pdf (Note: It's free!)

Knudson, L. (2014). Reprocessing complex surgical instruments requires adherence to manufacturers' instructions. *AORN Journal, 99*(1), C1-C8.

Wells, M.S.W. (2013). Elimination of immediate-use sterilization of radioactive seed implants. *AORN Journal, 97*(5), 515-520.

Module 3: Packaging and Sterilization of Instruments and Supplies

Introduction

The choice of packaging for instruments and supplies to be delivered to the sterile field is contingent on the item to be sterilized and the method of sterilization. Steam sterilization is the oldest, safest, most economical, and best understood method of sterilization; however, low temperature sterilization is becoming more popular for items that are moisture or heat sensitive.

Immediate use steam sterilization (IUSS) (previously call "flash sterilization") refers to steam sterilizing unwrapped items using an abbreviated (no drying time) cycle for immediate use on the sterile field. IUSS is intended for emergency situations only, such as accidental contamination of an item when no replacement is available. However, IUSS is frequently used to decrease turnaround time and as an alternative to increasing inventory. Neither of these uses of IUSS is acceptable. The Joint Commission and regulatory agencies have developed strict guidelines for immediate use sterilization. These guidelines are reflected in AORN's *Perioperative Standards and Recommended Practices*.

Competency Outcomes

To successfully complete the activities in this module, you will need to be able to:

1. Choose the correct method of sterilization for surgical instrumentation.
2. Describe processes for packaging an item for sterilization.

Recommended Readings

Alexander's Care of the Patient in Surgery. (2015, 15th ed.), Chapter 4: Infection prevention and control; Chapter 8: Surgical modalities.

Berry and Kohn's Operating Room Technique. (2013, 12th ed.), Chapter 18: Sterilization.

Perioperative Standards and Recommended Practices. (2014), Recommended practices:
- Cleaning and care of instruments and powered equipment.
- Selection and use of packaging systems for sterilization.
- Sterilization.

Key Words

Dynamic air removal, gravity displacement, hydrogen peroxide gas plasma sterilization, immediate use steam sterilization, implants, load, prevacuum, steam, sterilization

Activity — Fill in the Blank

Complete the chart below for typical cycle times for *dynamic air removal (prevacuum)* steam sterilization.

Item	Exposure time at 270° F (132° C)	Minimum dry time	Exposure time at 275° F (135° C)	Minimum dry time
Packaged instruments	_____	_____	_____	_____
Textile packs	_____	_____	_____	_____

Complete the chart below for typical cycle times for *gravity displacement* steam sterilization.

Item	Exposure time at 250° F (121° C)	Minimum dry time	Exposure time at 270° F (132° C)	Minimum dry time	Exposure time at 275° F (135° C)	Minimum dry time
Packaged instruments	_____	_____	_____	_____	_____	_____
Textile packs	_____	_____	_____	_____	_____	_____

Activity — Critical Thinking

Use the autoclave tape on the right to answer the following question.

1. What method of sterilization is indicated in the printout?

2. What type(s) of instruments can be processed using this method of sterilization?

3. What type(s) of monitoring should be used for this method of sterilization?

4. Under what set of circumstances should this method of sterilization be used?

5. When is it inappropriate to use this method of sterilization?

6. How should this cycle be documented?

```
========================
=======P R E V A C======
========================
CYCLE  START  AT  10:53:06A
                  ON    4/06/11

CYCLE  COUNT       28827
OPERATOR _____
   STERLIZER      VAC  S2

     STER TEMP  =   270.0F
  CONTROL TEMP  =   273.0F
     STER TIME  =   4 MIN
      DRY TIME  =   0 MIN

                       V=inHg
- TIME          T=F    P=psig

C  10:53:06A    146.4    0P
C  10:54:05A    249.1   21P
C  10:55:19A    181.8   22V
C  10:55:39A    249.7   26P
C  10:56:59A    110.5   22V
C  10:57:15A    237.5   26P
C  10:58:31A    168.2   22V
C  10:58:46A    247.3   26P
C  11:00:02A    179.6   23V
S  11:00:40A    270.1   32P
S  11:02:40A    273.5   32P
E  11:04:40A    273.2   31P
E  11:04:55A    233.7    3P
E  11:04:56A    232.6    2P
Z  11:05:08A    207.3    0P

LOAD                  040602

   TEMP MAX  =  273.8F
   TEMP MIN  =  270.1F

CONDITION   = 7:34
STERILIZE   = 4:00
EXHAUST     = 0:29
TOTAL CYCLE = 12:03

========================
=    READY TO UNLOAD    =
========================

* NOT READY        3:22:48P
DOOR UNLOCKED
```

Activity — Short Answer

What special packaging requirement does low temperature hydrogen peroxide sterilization have?

Activity — Fill in the Blank

1. What microorganism is used in the biological monitor for steam sterilization?

   _____.

2. During sterilization of double paper-plastic pouch packages, the packages should be

   placed _____.
   (paper-to-paper or paper-to-plastic).

3. Which of the following sterilization methods is NOT considered low-temperature?
   ___Steam autoclave
   ___Hydrogen peroxide gas plasma
   ___Peracetic acid
   ___Ozone

Additional Readings/Resources

AAMI. (2013). *Comprehensive Guide to Steam Sterilization and Sterility Assurance in Healthcare Facilities.* (ANSI/AAMI ST79: 2010/ A4:2013). Arlington, VA.: AAMI.

AAMI. *Immediate-Use Steam Sterilization.* Retrieved Feb. 18, 2014, from http://www.aami.org/publications/standards/ST79_Immediate_Use_Statement.pdf.

Centers for Disease Control and Prevention. (2008). *Guideline for Disinfection and Sterilization in Healthcare Facilities.* Retrieved Feb. 18, 2014, from http://www.cdc.gov/hicpac/Disinfection_Sterilization/toc.html (Note: It's free!)

Huber, L. (2010). Central sterile supply department professionals: A key piece in the OR quality puzzle. *AORN Journal, 91*(3), 319-320.

Huter-Kunish, G.G. (2009). Processing loaner instruments in an ambulatory surgery center. *AORN Journal, 89*(5), 861-870.

Hutzler, L., Kraemer, K., Iaboni, L., et al. (2013). A hospital-wide initiative to eliminate preventable causes of immediate use steam sterilization. *AORN Journal, 98*(6), 597-607.

Lucas, A. D., Chobin, N., Conner, R., Gordon E. A., et al. (2009). Steam sterilization and internal count sheets: Assessing the potential for cytotoxicity. *AORN Journal, 89*(3), 521-531.

Moore, T.K. (2009). Today's sterilizer is not your father's water heater. *AORN Journal, 90*(1), 81-92.

Morris, M. L. (2011). Sterilization in the perioperative setting. *AORN Journal, 93*(3), 411-412.

Nania, P. (2013). Immediate use steam sterilization: It's all about the process. *AORN Journal, 98*(1), 32-38.

Seavey, R. (2010). Collaboration between perioperative nurses and sterile processing personnel. *AORN Journal, 91*(4), 454-462.

Stanton, C. (2009). Staying current on sterilization standards. *AORN Journal, 90*(6), S114-S115.

Module 4: Principles of Transporting and Storing Sterile Supplies

Introduction

Instrumentation may be appropriately cleaned, decontaminated, disinfected, packaged, and sterilized, and still arrive at the sterile field contaminated. Transporting and storing instruments safely from the point of processing to the point of use requires the same attention to detail as any other step in the process.

Competency Outcomes

To successfully complete the activities in this module, you will need to be able to:

1. Identify safe storage principles for surgical instrumentation.
2. Select correct methods for transporting sterile supplies.

Recommended Readings

Alexander's Care of the Patient in Surgery. (2015, 15th ed.), Chapter 4: Infection prevention and control.

Berry and Kohn's Operating Room Technique. (2013, 12th ed.), Chapter 18: Sterilization.

Perioperative Standards and Recommended Practices. (2014), Recommended practices:
• Cleaning and care of instruments and powered equipment.
• Cleaning and processing endoscopes.
• Selection and use of packaging systems for sterilization.
• Sterilization.

Key Words

Controlled conditions, event related, shelf life, storage, time related, transportation

Activity — Know Your Numbers

Sterile items should be stored at least _____ inches above the floor, at least _____

inches below sprinkler heads, and at least _____ inches from outside walls.

Activity — Short Answer

What influences the shelf life of a packaged sterile item?

Activity — Multiple Choice

A flexible endoscope should be high-level disinfected before use if it has been unused for

    A. one day.
    B. three days.
    C. five days.
    D. it is not necessary for endoscopes to be high-level disinfected.

Activity — Critical Thinking

You send an orderly to pick up a pacemaker battery that has just been delivered to the receiving area of central services. The battery is in a sealed, sterile package and is still in its cardboard shipping carton. You are busy, so the orderly places the carton on a prep table inside the room.

What action should be taken?

Case Study Activity

Your scrub person has requested another drill. You bring in the rigid instrument tray and open it appropriately on a small table. As you remove the lid to the instrument tray, you notice beads of water on the inside of the tray. The process indicator shows that it has been exposed to the sterilization cycle. The tray was in its customary location in the sterile supply room.

1. Can the drill be considered sterile?

2. What are your options?

3. What is the significance of the load cycle lot number in this instance?

Additional Readings/Resources

Blanchard, J. (2009). Humidity, temperature, and air exchanges in the OR. *AORN Journal, 89*(6), 1129-1131.

Denholm, B. (2009). CMS requirements for sterile storage expiration dates in ASCs. *AORN Journal, 89*(5), 914-916.

Module 5: Principles of Biological and Chemical Monitoring

Introduction

Multiple methods are available for ensuring that instruments have been exposed to an environment conducive to destroying microorganisms. Biological and chemical integrators provide other quality assurance indicators that sterile instruments are being delivered to the surgical field.

Competency Outcomes

To successfully complete the activities in this module, you will need to be able to:

1. Differentiate between physical, chemical, and biological indicators.
2. Identify appropriate uses for Class 1, 2, 3, 4, 5, and 6 indicators.
3. Evaluate sterilization monitoring practices.

Recommended Readings

Alexander's Care of the Patient in Surgery. (2015, 15th ed.), Chapter 4: Infection prevention and control.

Berry and Kohn's Operating Room Technique. (2013, 12th ed.), Chapter 18: Sterilization.

Perioperative Standards and Recommended Practices. (2014), Recommended practices:
• Selection and use of packaging systems for sterilization.
• Sterilization.

Key Words

Biological indicator, Bowie-Dick dynamic air removal test, chemical indicator, emulating indicator, integrating indicator, pressure, process indicator, temperature

Activity — Do You Know?

What is the figure to the right?

What is its purpose?

How is it used?

Was the test successful or not?

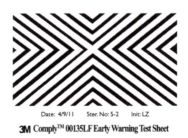

Date: 4/9/11   Ster. No: 5-2   Init: LZ

3M Comply™ 00135LF Early Warning Test Sheet

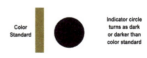

Color Standard

Indicator circle turns as dark or darker than color standard

Activity — Matching

Match the indicator to its definition.

Class 1 _____

Class 2 _____

Class 3 _____

Class 4 _____

Class 5 _____

Class 6 _____

Physical monitor _____

Biological indicator _____

A. time, pressure, temperature readout

B. single-variable indicator

C. used to monitor every implant load

D. used on outside of every package

E. Bowie-Dick dynamic air removal test

F. multi-variable indicator

G. integrating indicator (reacts to all critical parameters)

H. emulating indicator (reacts to all critical parameters of a specified sterilization cycle)

Activity — Critical Thinking

You are the circulator opening a set of instruments for an open reduction and internal fixation of a left ankle. There are three trays of specialty instrumentation, including implantable plates and screws for this procedure. All trays are labeled and identified with the same load number. All indicator tapes outside of the wrapped trays have turned color, indicating steam exposure. One of the trays does not have a chemical indicator inside of the tray. The other two have chemical indicators that have turned color, indicating effective steam penetration. The case is scheduled to begin in 30 minutes.

1. Can you assume that the instrumentation is sterile based on the two trays having positive indicators and being from the same cycle of the sterilizer?

2. What are your options? What are the pros and cons of each?

3. How could this situation be avoided in the future?

Additional Readings/Resources

Chard, R. (2009). Tracking sterilization loads that contain implants. *AORN Journal, 90*(1), 117.

Mitchell, S. (2009). Class 6 emulating chemical indicators and process challenge packs. *AORN Journal, 90*(2), 279-280.

Module 6: Safe Handling Practices for Hazardous and Biohazardous Materials

Introduction

Any substance that poses a health threat to people or the environment requires special care in both handling and disposition. Perioperative nurses are responsible for ensuring that the work environment is safe for patients, fellow workers, and themselves.

Competency Outcomes

To successfully complete the activities in this module, you will need to be able to:

1. Identify potential sources of injury to personnel in the perioperative setting.
2. Employ methods for maintaining a safe environment.

Recommended Readings

Alexander's Care of the Patient in Surgery. (2015, 15th ed.), Chapter 3: Workplace issues and staff safety.

Berry and Kohn's Operating Room Technique. (2013, 12th ed.), Chapter 13: Potential sources of injury to the caregiver and the patient.

Perioperative Standards and Recommended Practices. (2014), Recommended practices for safe environment of care.

Key Words

Anesthesia waste gases, bloodborne pathogen, chemotherapy, hands-free zone, methyl methacrylate, MSDS, neutral zone, sharps safety, smoke plume

Activity — Short Answer

What are the four major ways to reduce needlestick injuries in the perioperative setting?

1. _____

2. _____

3. _____

4. _____

Activity — Critical Thinking

Is a smoke evacuation system needed for laparoscopic procedures? Explain your response.

Case Study Activity

What practices should be implemented to limit exposure of methyl methacrylate to OR personnel?

Activity — Multiple Choice

What is the *best* way to dispose of unused chemotherapy agents?

A. Flush them down the hopper.

B. Place in impervious container and send with patient.

C. Follow federal, state, and local laws in consultation with health care organization's pharmacist.

D. Place them in a hazardous transport container and dispose of it with other OR waste.

E. Follow OSHA guidelines.

Additional Readings/Resources

Hart, P.B. (2011). Bloodborne pathogen violations: Compliance is key to prevention. *AORN Journal, 94*(5), 480-487.

Lucas, A.D., Chobin, N., Conner, R., et al. (2009). Steam sterilization and internal count sheets: Assessing the potential for cytotoxicity. *AORN Journal, 89*(3), 521-531.

Mellinger, E., Skinker, L., Sears, D., Gardner, D., et al. (2010). Safe handling of chemotherapy in the perioperative setting. *AORN Journal, 91*(4), 435-453.

National Institute for Occupational Safety and Health (NIOSH). (2004). Preventing occupational exposures to antineoplastic and other hazardous drugs in health care settings. NIOSH Alert (Pub no. 2004-165).Washington, DC. Retrieved Feb. 18, 2014, from http://www.cdc.gov/niosh/docs/2004-165/

Vose, J.G., & McAdara-Berkowitz, J. (2009). Reducing scalpel injuries in the operating room. *AORN Journal, 98*(6), 867-872.

Willemson-McBride, T.L. (2009). Safe handling of cytotoxic agents: A team approach. *AORN Journal, 90*(5), 731-740.

"Go To" Activity — Skill Building

Locate the MSDS reference in your department.

Talk with your risk mitigation manager or infection prevention specialist about your facility's exposure control plan.

Chapter Summary

Sterility is the hallmark of the operating room; it is the one defining characteristic that makes the environment safe for surgery. Your knowledge and application of the principles and practice of disinfection and sterilization have a direct impact on patient safety. The disinfection and sterilization of instruments begin at the point of use — when a sterile instrument is delivered to the sterile field. Though we may not initially process the instruments and equipment, we are accountable to our patients for delivering the safest possible patient care.

Glossary

Airborne precautions — Precautions used when caring for patients with known or suspected microorganisms that can be transmitted by the airborne route.

Aseptic technique — Practices that restrict microorganisms in the environment and on equipment and supplies and that prevent normal body flora from contaminating the surgical wound.

Association for the Advancement of Medical Instrumentation (AAMI) — Alliance of health care professions dedicated to increasing the understanding, safety, and efficacy of medical instrumentation.

Bioburden — Amount of microbial load on an item before sterilization.

Biohazardous waste — Contaminated with blood, body fluids, or tissues capable of transmitting infection.

Biological indicator — A sterilization process monitoring device containing a known population of highly resistant spores that is used to test the effectiveness of sterilization.

Chemical indicator — A device used to monitor the attainment of one or more critical parameters of the sterilization cycle. A characteristic color change indicates a defined level of exposure based on the conditions within the sterilization chamber.

Cleaning — Using friction, detergent, and water to remove soil and debris. Cleaning removes, rather than kills, microorganisms.

Contact precautions — Precautions designed to reduce the risk of transmission of infectious microorganisms transmitted by direct or indirect contact.

Critical item — Item that contacts the vascular system or enters sterile tissue or body cavities; poses the highest risk for transmission of infection.

Decontamination — Cleaning and disinfecting or sterilizing processes carried out to make contaminated items safe to handle.

Disinfection — The process of eliminating many or all pathogenic organisms except bacterial spores from inanimate objects.

Droplet precautions — Precautions used when caring for patients with known or suspected microorganisms that can be transmitted by infectious large particle (i.e., 5 microns or larger) droplets.

Dynamic air removal (pre-vacuum and steam-flush pressure-pulse steam sterilizers) — Incorporates mechanically assisted air removal from the sterilization chamber.

Emulating indicators (Class 6) — Chemical indicators (CIs) designed to change color when exposed to critical variables (time, temperature, and the presence of steam) for a specified sterilization cycle. Because they are not required to correlate to performance of biological indicators (BIs), Class 6 CIs are not recommended in place of BIs in load monitoring.

Enzymatic cleaner — Cleaning agent that uses enzymes to remove protein from surgical instruments.

Event related — Factors that may influence the shelf life of a sterilized item, such as excessive handling or humidity. Shelf life is based on the premise that items have been properly cleaned, decontaminated, wrapped or containerized, stored, and handled.

Food and Drug Administration (FDA) — An agency of the U.S. Department of Health and Human Services, responsible for protecting and promoting public health through the regulation and supervision of medical devices.

Germicide — A disinfectant that kills pathogenic microorganisms.

Gravity displacement — A type of steam sterilization cycle in which incoming air displaces residual air through a port or drain near the bottom of the sterilizer chamber.

Hazardous waste — Any substance that poses a health threat to persons or the environment.

High-level disinfection — Process that kills all microorganisms with the exception of high numbers of bacterial spores and prions. Inactivates *Mycobacterium tuberculosis*, Hepatitis B, HIV, vegetative bacteria, and some spores and fungi. It is not effective against prions that cause Creutzfeld-Jacob disease.

Immediate use steam sterilization (IUSS, previously known as "flash" sterilization) — Sterilization of unwrapped items at point of use for a specific patient or procedure, using an abbreviated sterilization cycle.

Integrating indicators (Class 5) — Chemical indicators (CIs) designed to reach their endpoint response when exposed to critical variables (time, temperature, and the presence of steam). This CI provides the most thorough information about the effectiveness of steam sterilization cycles.

Intermediate-level disinfection — Level of disinfection that kills *Mycobacterium tuberculosis*, vegetative bacteria, most viruses, and most fungi, but does not necessarily kill bacterial spores.

Loaner instrumentation — Borrowed or consigned surgical instruments, equipment, and supplies brought in from outside the facility.

Low-level disinfection — Level of disinfection that kills most bacteria, some viruses, and some fungi. It cannot be relied on to kill resistant organisms or spores.

Non-critical item — Item that comes in contact with intact skin but not with mucous membranes, sterile tissue, or the vascular system.

Pathogen — Any microorganism capable of causing disease.

Personal protective equipment (PPE) — Specialized equipment or supplies (gown, gloves, mask, eye protection, etc.) used to protect the worker from injury or exposure to environmental hazards.

Prion — Infectious protein particle responsible for transmissible spongiform encephalopathies (i.e., Creutzfeld-Jacob disease in humans).

Semi-critical item — Item that comes in contact with mucous membranes or non-intact skin.

Shelf life — Length of time an item is safe to use.

Spaulding classification — Recommended methods for disinfection and sterilization of items based on whether the item encounters intact skin, mucous membranes, sterile tissue, or the vascular system.

Standard precautions — Precautions used in the care of all patients, regardless of known or suspected disease processes. As used in the Job Analysis, this term refers to the standard and transmission-based precautions policies and procedures as developed by the CDC and OSHA.

Sterilization — Process that kills all living microorganisms (bacteria, fungi, virus, and bacterial spores).

Surgical conscience/sterile conscience — Awareness that develops from a keen understanding of the importance of strict adherence to principles of aseptic technique.

Transmission-based precautions — Practices for patients with specific or suspected infectious processes with highly transmissible or epidemiologically important pathogens. Includes airborne, droplet, and contact precautions.

References

AORN. (2014). *Perioperative Standards and Recommended Practices*. Denver: AORN, Inc.

Centers for Disease Control and Prevention (CDC). Healthcare-associated infections. Retrieved Feb. 18, 2014, from http://www.cdc.gov/HAI/ssi/ssi.html

Centers for Disease Control and Prevention (CDC). (1999, April). Guideline for prevention of surgical site infections. *Infection Control and Hospital Epidemiology*, 20(4), 247-279. Retrieved April 28, 2014, from http://www.cdc.gov/hicpac/pdf/guidelines/ SSI_1999.pdf

Phillips, N. (2013). *Berry and Kohn's Operating Room Technique* (12th ed.). St. Louis: Mosby.

Rothrock, J.C. (Ed.). (2015). *Alexander's Care of the Patient in Surgery* (15th ed.). St. Louis: Mosby.

Answers to Chapter 6 Activities

Module 1: Microbiological considerations related to infection control principles — Pages 176-179

Activity — Fill in the Blank

What is considered the most important and effective intervention for preventing infections?

Hand hygiene.

> Source: Rothrock, J.C. (Ed.). (2015). *Alexander's Care of the Patient in Surgery* (15th ed., p. 83). St. Louis: Mosby.

Activity — Stop the Spread! Part 1

For each of the following diseases, choose the appropriate transmission-based precautions.

Human immunodeficiency virus (HIV): *A*

Mycobacterium tuberculosis: *C*

Hepatitis B: *A*

Staphylococcus aureus: *A*

Clostridium difficile: *A*

Pseudomonas: *A*

Varicella: *C*

Influenza: *B*

A. Contact

B. Droplet

A. Airborne

Activity — Stop the Spread! Part 2

Draw a line between each type of precaution and its appropriate method of preventing transmission. Use each answer only once.

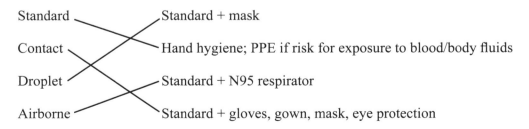

Standard — Standard + mask

Contact — Hand hygiene; PPE if risk for exposure to blood/body fluids

Droplet — Standard + N95 respirator

Airborne — Standard + gloves, gown, mask, eye protection

> Source: AORN. (2014). Recommended practices: Prevention of transmissible infections. In *Perioperative Standards and Recommended Practices*, pp. 386, 388-392, 404. Denver: AORN, Inc.

Activity — Critical Thinking

You have just cared for a patient who is suspected of having Creutzfeld-Jacob disease (CJD). What is the preferred method for inactivating prions on semi-critical and critical devices exposed to high-infectivity tissue?

Gravity steam sterilization for 30 minutes at 131° C (268° F) or dynamic air removal steam sterilization for 18 minutes at 134° C to 138° C (273° F to 280° F).

Source: AORN. (2014). Recommended practices for cleaning and care of surgical instruments and powered equipment. In *Perioperative Standards and Recommended Practices*, p. 517. Denver: AORN, Inc.

Case Study Activity

In evaluating Mr. J., what risk factors for a surgical site infection do you find?

Age, Implants, Elevated WBCs signifying possible pre-existing infection, Steroid use

Source: Phillips, N. (2013). *Berry and Kohn's Operating Room Technique* (12th ed., p. 237). St. Louis: Mosby.

Module 2: Cleaning and disinfecting instruments and supplies — Pages 180-184

Activity — Multiple Choice

Circle the most reliable source for information regarding processing of instruments and equipment:
   A. OSHA regulations
   B. TJC requirements
   C. FDA protocols
   D. Manufacturers' instructions

D. Manufacturers' instructions

Source: AORN. (2014). Recommended practices for cleaning and care of surgical instruments and powered equipment. In *Perioperative Standards and Recommended Practices*, p. 541. Denver: AORN, Inc.

Activity — Matching

Match the item to its definition.

1. Non-critical - *C*	A. Enters sterile tissues including the vascular system
2. Semi-critical - *B*	B. Contacts non-intact skin and mucous membranes
3. Critical - *A*	C. Contacts intact skin or does not come in contact with the patient

Source: AORN. (2014). Recommended practices for high-level disinfection. In *Perioperative Standards and Recommended Practices*, pp. 515-516. Denver: AORN, Inc.

Activity — Put It In Its Place

Match the following items to the potential for transmitting infection and their appropriate method of processing.

Disease transmission risk	Item	Method of processing
Non-critical	***Blood pressure cuff*** ***Tourniquet cuff*** ***Doppler*** ***Mayo stand***	Intermediate-level disinfection
Semi-critical	***Laryngoscope*** ***Colonoscope***	High-level disinfection
Critical	***Balfour retractor*** ***Urinary catheter***	Sterilization

Source: AORN. (2014). Recommended practices for high-level disinfection. In *Perioperative Standards and Recommended Practices*, p. 516. Denver: AORN, Inc.

Activity — Do You Know?

Check all of the following that represent proper management of instruments used during a surgical procedure:

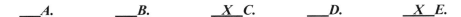

___*A.*   ___*B.*   _*X*_*C.*   ___*D.*   _*X*_*E.*

Source: AORN. (2014). Recommended practices for care of instruments. In *Perioperative Standards and Recommended Practices*, pp. 542-544. Denver: AORN, Inc.

Activity — Scramble

Number the following steps in high-level disinfection in the correct order:

5 - Flush lumens with disinfectant.
3 - Clean the instrument.
6 - Time the immersion cycle.
1 - Wear appropriate PPE.
9 - Document results of processing.
2 - Check solution for minimum effective concentration.
8 - Deliver to point of use without contaminating.
7 - Rinse with sterile water.
4 - Immerse instrument in disinfectant according to manufacturer's recommendations.

Source: AORN. (2014). Recommended practices for high-level disinfection. In *Perioperative Standards and Recommended Practices*, pp. 519-521. Denver: AORN, Inc.

Activity — Short Answer

How long can an item that has been high-level disinfected be stored before use?

Items that are high-level disinfected must be used immediately.

   Source: AORN. (2014). Recommended practices for high-level disinfection. In *Perioperative Standards and Recommended Practices*, p. 521. Denver: AORN, Inc.

Activity — Critical Thinking

A surgical instrumentation vendor arrives at 0715 for your scheduled 0730 anterior/posterior spinal fusion case with a set of implants. The implants have been sterilized at another facility and are covered with a heavy plastic dust cover. What is your response?

Loaner instrumentation should be examined, cleaned, and sterilized by the receiving health care organization before use. This case is not emergent, so immediate use sterilization should not be considered.

   Source: AORN. (2014). Recommended practices for cleaning and care of instruments. In *Perioperative Standards and Recommended Practices*, p. 542. Denver: AORN, Inc.

Module 3: Packaging and sterilization of instruments and supplies — Pages 184-188

Activity — Fill in the Blank

Complete the chart for typical cycle times for *dynamic air removal (prevacuum)* steam sterilization.

Item	Exposure time at 270° F (132° C)	Minimum dry time	Exposure time at 275° F (135° C)	Minimum dry time
Packaged instruments	*4 min.*	*20-30 min.*	*3 min.*	*16 min.*
Textile packs	*4 min.*	*5-20 min.*	*3 min.*	*3 min.*

   Source: AORN. (2014). Recommended practices for sterilization. In *Perioperative Standards and Recommended Practices*, p. 581. Denver: AORN, Inc.

Complete the chart for typical cycle times for *gravity displacement* steam sterilization.

Item	Exposure time at 250° F (121° C)	Minimum dry time	Exposure time at 270° F (132° C)	Minimum dry time	Exposure time at 275° F (135° C)	Minimum dry time
Packaged instruments	*30 min.*	*15-30 min.*	*15 min.*	*15-30 min.*	*NA*	*NA*
Textile packs	*30 min.*	*15 min.*	*25 min.*	*15 min.*	*10 min.*	*30 min.*

Source: AORN. (2014). Recommended practices for sterilization. In *Perioperative Standards and Recommended Practices*, p. 580. Denver: AORN, Inc.

Activity — Critical Thinking

Use the autoclave tape to the right to answer the following question:

1. What method of sterilization is indicated in the printout?

Dynamic air removal (prevacuum) steam sterilization, 4 minute cycle, immediate use

2. What type(s) of instruments can be processed using this method of sterilization?

Metal, porous, with lumens

3. What type(s) of monitoring should be used for this method of sterilization?

Class 5 or Class 6 chemical indicators with every load, plus a rapid-action biological indicator (BI) if implants are being sterilized (NOT recommended to sterilize implants using this method except in cases of emergency when no other option is available). The load should be quarantined until the results of the BI are available.

4. Under what set of circumstances should this method of sterilization be used?

Use of a rigid sterilization container designed for immediate-use sterilization; insufficient time to process by the preferred wrapped or container method. Items still must be properly decontaminated prior to sterilization. Packaging/wrappers/towels should not be used unless sterilizer is specifically designed for such. Items are to be used immediately.

```
=====================
======P R E V A C======
=====================
CYCLE  START  AT  10:53:06A
                ON    4/06/11

CYCLE  COUNT      28827
OPERATOR _____
  STERLIZER        VAC S2

        STER TEMP  =  270.0F
    CONTROL TEMP  =  273.0F
        STER TIME  =   4 MIN
        DRY TIME  =   0 MIN

                      V=inHg
-TIME          T=F  P=psig

C  10:53:06A    146.4    0P
C  10:54:05A    249.1   21P
C  10:55:19A    181.8   22V
C  10:55:39A    249.7   26P
C  10:56:59A    110.5   22V
C  10:57:15A    237.5   26P
C  10:58:31A    168.2   22V
C  10:58:46A    247.3   26P
C  11:00:02A    179.6   23V
S  11:00:40A    270.1   32P
S  11:02:40A    273.5   32P
E  11:04:40A    273.2   31P
E  11:04:55A    233.7    3P
E  11:04:56A    232.6    2P
Z  11:05:08A    207.3    0P

LOAD              040602

    TEMP MAX  =  273.8F
    TEMP MIN  =  270.1F

CONDITION    = 7:34
STERILIZE    = 4:00
EXHAUST      = 0:29
TOTAL CYCLE  = 12:03

=====================
=    READY TO UNLOAD    =
=====================
* NOT READY          3:22:48P
DOOR UNLOCKED
```

5. When is it inappropriate to use this method of sterilization?

As a substitute for insufficient inventory; late arrival of loaner instrumentation and implantable devices; and when items will not be used immediately.

6. How should this cycle be documented?

Autoclave identification number, date, time, load number, type of sterilizer/cycle, contents of load, cycle parameters checked (e.g., temperature, duration of cycle), results of process monitoring indicators, operator, patient, and reason for immediate use sterilization.

Source: AORN. (2014). Recommended practices for sterilization. In *Perioperative Standards and Recommended Practices*, pp. 581-583. Denver: AORN, Inc.

Activity — Short Answer

What special packaging requirement does low temperature hydrogen peroxide sterilization have?

Hydrogen peroxide is incompatible with cellulose and will cause the load to abort; hence, no paper or linen can be used for packaging.

Source: Rothrock, J.C. (Ed.). (2015). *Alexander's Care of the Patient in Surgery* (15th ed., p. 98). St. Louis: Mosby.

Activity — Fill in the Blank

1. What microorganism is used in the biologic monitor for steam sterilization?

Geobacillus stearothermophilus

Source: AORN. (2014). Recommended practices for sterilization. In *Perioperative Standards and Recommended Practices*, p. 595. Denver: AORN, Inc.

2. During sterilization of double paper-plastic pouch packages, the packages should be placed

paper-to-paper

Source: AORN. (2014). Recommended practices for packaging systems. In *Perioperative Standards and Recommended Practices*, p. 567. Denver: AORN, Inc.

3. Which of the following sterilization methods is NOT considered low-temperature?

Steam autoclave

Source: Rothrock, J.C. (Ed.). (2015). *Alexander's Care of the Patient in Surgery* (15th ed., pp. 93, 96). St. Louis: Mosby.

Module 4: Principles of transporting and storing sterile supplies — Pages 188-190

Activity — Know Your Numbers

Sterile items should be stored at least *8-10* inches above the floor, at least *18* inches below sprinkler heads, and at least *2* inches from outside walls.

> Source: AORN. (2014). Recommended practices for sterilization. In *Perioperative Standards and Recommended Practices*, p. 591. Denver: AORN, Inc.

Activity — Short Answer

What influences the shelf life of a packaged sterile item?

Shelf life is determined by any factor that can alter the integrity of the packaging, such as amount of handling of the package and humidity of the storage room.

> Source: AORN. (2014). Recommended practices for selection and use of packaging systems. In *Perioperative Standards and Recommended Practices*, p. 564. Denver: AORN, Inc.

Activity — Multiple Choice

A flexible endoscope should be high-level disinfected before use if it has been unused for

C. five days.

> Source: AORN. (2014). Recommended practices for cleaning and processing endoscopes. In *Perioperative Standards and Recommended Practices*, p. 534. Denver: AORN, Inc.

Activity — Critical Thinking

You send an orderly to pick up a pacemaker battery that has just been delivered to the receiving area of central services. The battery is in a sealed, sterile package and is still in its cardboard shipping carton. You are busy, so the orderly places the carton on a prep table inside the room. What action should be taken?

The shipping carton should be immediately removed from the sterile area. It is a reservoir for dust and other contaminants. The prep table should be disinfected with a hospital-grade germicide. The orderly should be instructed on the appropriate way to transport sterile supplies in the OR.

> Source: AORN. (2014). Recommended practices for sterilization. In *Perioperative Standards and Recommended Practices*, p. 591. Denver: AORN, Inc.

Case Study Activity

Your scrub person has requested another drill. You bring in the rigid instrument tray and open it appropriately on a small table. As you remove the lid to the instrument tray, you notice beads of water on the inside of the tray. The process indicator shows that it has been exposed to the sterilization cycle. The tray was in its customary location in the sterile supply room.

1. Can the drill be considered sterile?

No. Wrapped instruments that are opened and found to be wet cannot be considered sterile.

2. What are your options?

The tray should be removed from the OR and a new sterile tray brought to the room. If immediate-use steam sterilization is necessary, the drill should be decontaminated appropriately first.

3. What is the significance of the load cycle lot number in this instance?

The load cycle lot number will need to be tracked to recall all other items in that load for possible wetness and contamination. Autoclave failure and corrective action will need to be documented and reported to OR and SPD managers, infection prevention, and quality assurance. If the sterilizer has malfunctioned, surgeons will need to be contacted with patient information.

Source: AORN. (2014). Recommended practices for sterilization. In *Perioperative Standards and Recommended Practices*, pp. 581-583; 593-595. Denver: AORN, Inc.

Module 5: Principles of biological and chemical monitoring — Pages 191-193

Activity — Do You Know?

What is the figure to the right? What is its purpose? How is it used? Was the test successful or not?

This is a chemical indicator Class 2 Bowie-Dick air removal test. It is used to detect residual air in the dynamic air-removal sterilizer. The graph is wrapped in the center of a test pack and placed on the lower shelf of an empty sterilizer chamber. The sterilizer is then run. It is used to measure the efficacy of the air removal system, not sterility. This test is a "pass."

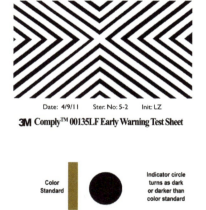

Date: 4/9/11   Ster. No: 5-2   Init: LZ

3M Comply™ 00135LF Early Warning Test Sheet

Color Standard

Indicator circle turns as dark or darker than color standard

Source: AORN. (2014). Recommended practices for sterilization. In *Perioperative Standards and Recommended Practices*, pp. 596-597. Denver: AORN, Inc.

Activity — Matching

Match the indicator to its definition.

Class 1 - **D**
Class 2 - **E**
Class 3 - **B**
Class 4 - **F**
Class 5 - **G**
Class 6 - **H**
Physical monitor - **A**
Biological indicator - **C**

A. time, pressure, temperature readout
B. single-variable indicator
C. used to monitor every implant load
D. used on outside of every package
E. Bowie-Dick dynamic air removal test
F. multi-variable indicator
G. integrating indicator (reacts to all critical parameters)
H. emulating indicator (reacts to all critical parameters of a specified sterilization cycle)

Source: AORN. (2014). Recommended practices for sterilization. In *Perioperative Standards and Recommended Practices*, p. 571. Denver: AORN, Inc.

Activity — Critical Thinking

You are the circulator opening a set of instruments for an open reduction and internal fixation of a left ankle. There are three trays of specialty instrumentation, including implantable plates and screws for this procedure. All trays are labeled and identified with the same load number. All indicator tapes outside of the wrapped trays have turned color, indicating steam exposure. One of the trays does not have a chemical indicator inside of the tray. The other two have chemical indicators that have turned color, indicating effective steam penetration. The case is scheduled to begin in 30 minutes.

1. Can you assume that the instrumentation is sterile based on the two trays having positive indicators and being from the same cycle of the sterilizer?

You cannot assume that the instrumentation is sterile based on the results of the other trays from the same cycle of the same sterilizer. There is no definitive way to determine that steam reached the inner contents of the tray without an indicator.

2. What are your options? What are the pros and cons of each?

Is a sterile replacement tray available? If not, then the choices are:
- *Delaying the case may present an inconvenience to the patient and surgical team. However, appropriate processing of the instrumentation to provide sterile implants takes precedence and will help ensure optimal results for the patient.*
- *Immediate-use steam sterilization (IUSS), previously known as "flash sterilization," is not recommended for any instrumentation, including implantable devices (e.g., plates and screws). If this option is chosen, a rapid-action biological indicator as well as a chemical indicator must be used, and the instruments must be quarantined until the results are read. The risk of contamination increases with IUSS because of the additional handling required to transport the tray from the sterilizer to the field.*

3. How could this situation be avoided in the future?

Planning and coordination will alleviate the need for flash sterilization. This includes scheduling cases appropriately (e.g., not scheduling cases requiring the same instrumentation back-to-

back) and ensuring adequate numbers of instruments are available to perform multiple cases without flash sterilizing instruments. Notify sterile processing department of incident.

Source: AORN. (2014). Recommended practices for sterilization. In *Perioperative Standards and Recommended Practices*, pp. 579-583. Denver: AORN, Inc.

Module 6: Safe handling practices for hazardous and biohazardous materials — Pages 193-195

Activity — Short Answer

What are the four major ways to reduce needlestick injuries in the perioperative setting?

Engineered sharps injury protection devices
Double gloving
Neutral zone
Blunt suture needles

Source: AORN. (2014). Recommended practices for sharps safety. In *Perioperative Standards and Recommended Practices*, p. 352. Denver: AORN, Inc.

Activity — Critical Thinking

Is a smoke evacuation system needed for laparoscopic procedures? Explain your response.

Surgical smoke should be evacuated and filtered during laparoscopic procedures. Smoke contained in the peritoneum may be more concentrated than that released during an open procedure. Although the risk to the patient is unknown, the concentrated smoke released directly from the cannula can expose the peioperative team to contaminants.

Source: AORN. (2014). Recommended practices for minimally invasive surgery. In *Perioperative Standards and Recommended Practices*, p. 166. Denver: AORN, Inc.

Activity — Case Study

What practices should be implemented to limit exposure of methyl methacrylate to OR personnel?

- *Methods for reducing fumes (e.g., vacuum mixer, activated charcoal).*
- *Protective eyewear.*
- *Follow manufacturers' recommendations for mixing and required PPEs.*
- *Double glove.*
- *Use cement gun or mixing system to avoid contact with cement until it is the consistency of dough.*
- *Dispose of as a hazardous waste.*

Source: AORN. (2014). Recommended practices for a safe environment of care. In *Perioperative Standards and Recommended Practices*, pp. 243-245. Denver: AORN, Inc.

Activity — Multiple Choice

What is the *best* way to dispose of unused chemotherapy agents?

C. Follow federal, state, and local laws in consultation with health care organization's pharmacist.

Source: AORN. (2014). Recommended practices for a safe environment of care, pp. 245-246; Recommended practices for medication safety. In *Perioperative Standards and Recommended Practices*, pp. 297-298. Denver: AORN, Inc.

NOTES

CHAPTER 7:
Emergency Situations

> **Test Specifications:**
> **8% of CNOR test questions are based on Emergency Situations.**

Introduction

The actions of the perioperative nurse in emergencies, regardless of the nature of the situation, are comparable to his or her responses during all patient care activities with the exception of time. There are two types of intraoperative emergencies: those that contributed to the need for the surgery, and those that emerge during the procedure itself. Both situations require clinical competence, critical thinking, speed of decision making, the ability to organize resources, and good communication skills.

Regardless of the nature of the emergency, the goals for treatment are:
1. Maintenance of an open airway.
2. Maintenance of circulating blood volume.
3. Perfusion of oxygen to vital organs to support function.

This chapter will help you review common emergencies and the appropriate nursing interventions necessary to successfully manage them. Anticipating and preventing emergencies by recognizing and treating early warning signs are emphasized.

Module 1: Anaphylaxis

Anaphylaxis is a life-threatening allergic reaction involving multiple organ systems. Anaphylaxis occuring during the perioperative period is most commonly associated with blood transfusions, muscle relaxants, latex, antibiotics, and anesthetic agents. Because death from cardiovascular collapse can occur quickly, prevention is always the best nursing intervention. The first step in prevention lies in taking a complete and accurate patient assessment.

Competency Outcomes

To successfully complete the activities in this module, you will need to be able to:

1. Describe the signs and symptoms of anaphylaxis.
2. Discuss nursing interventions for the patient experiencing an allergic reaction.

Recommended Readings

Alexander's Care of the Patient in Surgery. (2015, 15th ed.), pp. 38, 64-65, 113.

Berry and Kohn's Operating Room Technique. (2013, 12th.), pp. 230-231, 248, 632.

Perioperative Standards and Recommended Practices. (2014), Recommended practices for a safe environment of care.

Key Words

Allergy, anaphylactic shock, anaphylaxis, latex free, latex safe, sensitivity, transfusion reaction

Activity — Critical Thinking

You are assigned to care for Mrs. M., who has been diagnosed with a latex allergy. She is scheduled as the third case of the day. Describe your plan to decrease Mrs. M.'s risk for developing a latex reaction during her perioperative experience.

Activity — Do You Know?

Number the following interventions for a suspected blood transfusion reaction in the appropriate order.

____ Send a sample of the patient's urine to the lab.
____ Complete an occurrence/incident report.
____ Stop the transfusion.
____ Document and communicate reaction, interventions, and patient responses to the next caregiver.
____ Anticipate orders for emergency drugs.
____ Monitor the patient carefully.
____ Return unused blood, tubing, and a sample of the patient's blood to the blood bank.
____ Replace IV tubing and hang 0.9% sodium chloride.
____ Report reaction to surgeon and blood bank.

Activity — Critical Thinking

Many of the signs and symptoms of a blood transfusion reaction (e.g., chills, backache, shivering) are masked by a general anesthetic. How could you tell if your patient under a general anesthetic is having an adverse reaction to a blood transfusion?

Additional Readings/Resources

Briesemeister, E., & Burlingame, B.L. (2006). Shellfish and iodine allergies. *AORN Journal, 83*(2), 479.

Bundesen, I-M. (2008). Natural rubber latex: A matter of concern for nurses. *AORN Journal, 88*(2), 197-210.

Girard, N. (2011). Transfusion "slip". *AORN Journal, 94*(2), 216, 189.

Nelson, J. (2009). Latex in the perioperative setting: Strategies for patient and staff member safety. *AORN Journal, 89*(6), 1152.

"Go To" Activity — Skill Building

Identify and locate an acceptable alternative to any latex-containing supplies in your department.

Review your department's policy and procedure on providing a latex free environment for your patients.

Discuss with your department manager or educator about developing or updating a latex free item list for posting in surgical suites and sterile processing department.

Norred, C.L (2012). Anesthetic-induced anaphylaxis. *AANA Journal, 80*(2), 129-140. Retrieved Feb. 15, 2014, from http://www.aana.com/newsandjournal/Documents/jcourse1-0412-p129-140.pdf

Module 2: Cardiovascular Emergencies

Cardiac arrest is the leading cause of morbidity and mortality related to the surgical experience. Cardiac emergencies may arise from respiratory insufficiency or arrest, such as that seen in inadequate ventilation, pulmonary emboli, or hypoxia; complications related to the surgical intervention, such as blood loss, hypotension, dysrhythmias, or shock; or as a response to a disease process that has been exacerbated by the stress of surgery. Basic and advanced life-support skills must be implemented very quickly to help ensure a positive outcome for the patient.

Competency Outcomes

To successfully complete the activities in this module, you will need to be able to:

1. Identify common intraoperative cardiac emergencies.
2. Choose appropriate nursing interventions in managing the patient in cardiac arrest.

Recommended Readings

Alexander's Care of the Patient in Surgery. (2015, 15th ed.), pp. 231, 275-276, 279-280; Chapter 24: Vascular surgery; Chapter 25: Cardiac surgery.

Berry and Kohn's Operating Room Technique. (2013, 12th ed.), Chapter 31: Potential perioperative complications (pp. 611-624).

Key Words

Advanced cardiac life support, autologous blood, blood loss, cardiac arrest, cardiopulmonary resuscitation, circulating blood volume, circulation, deep vein thrombosis, dysrhythmia, embolus, fluid replacement, hemorrhage, hypertension, hypotension, shock, thrombus, transfusion

Activity — Short Answer

You are monitoring an 83-year-old man who is having a lesion removed from his back under local anesthetic. His pulse and respirations are being assessed manually. He is in the prone position. He complains of shortness of breath, and then chest pain. What actions should be initiated?

Additional Readings/Resources

Babb, M. (2009). Clinical risk assessment: Identifying patients at high risk for heart failure. *AORN Journal, 89*(2), 273-288.

Dobbenga-Rhodes, Y.A. (2009). Responding to amniotic fluid embolism. *AORN Journal, 89*(6), 1079-1092.

"Go To" Activity — Check It Out!

Go to Question #36, DIC, under the Perioperative question of the week tab in the Toolbox at http://www.cc-institute.org/toolbox for another critical-thinking activity.

Fisher, L. (2011). Perioperative care of the patient with sickle cell disease. *AORN Journal, 93*(1), 150-159.

Murdoch, D.B. (2013). Perioperative cardiopulmonary arrest competencies. *AORN Journal, 98*(2), 116-130.

Neveleff, D.J. (2012). Optimizing hemostatic practices: Matching the appropriate hemostat to the clinical situation. *AORN Journal, 96*(5), S1-S17.

Ozawa, S. (2013). Patient blood management: Use of topical hemostatic and sealant agents. *AORN Journal, 98*(5), 461-478.

Tinkham, M.R. (2009). The endovascular approach to abdominal aortic aneurysm repair. *AORN Journal, 89*(2), 289-306.

> ## "Go To" Activity — Skill Building
>
> Enroll in an EKG course offered by your facility or community college, or an on-line program.
>
> Review the contents of your department's CODE or COR cart. Are age-appropriate supplies available based on your patient population?
>
> Enroll in an ACLS course.
>
> Set up and participate in a mock COR for your department.

Module 3: Respiratory Complications

The first priority in any emergency is to obtain and maintain a patent airway. Assisting the anesthesia care provider takes priority over any other nursing duties.

Competency Outcomes

To successfully complete the activities in this module, you will need to be able to:
1. Identify common respiratory emergencies.
2. Apply appropriate nursing interventions to manage respiratory emergencies.

Recommended Readings

Alexander's Care of the Patient in Surgery. (2015, 15th ed.), pp. 140-143, 274-275, 279-280.

Berry and Kohn's Operating Room Technique. (2013, 12th ed.), Chapter 31: Potential perioperative complications (pp. 608-611).

Perioperative Standards and Recommended Practices. (2014), Recommended practices for managing the patient receiving moderate sedation/analgesia.

Key Words

Airway obstruction, anoxia, arterial blood gas, aspiration, atelectasis, bronchospasm, difficult airway, hypoxia, laryngospasm, pneumothorax, pulmonary edema, pulmonary embolism

Activity — Critical Thinking

You are the scrub person for a patient scheduled for a craniotomy. The patient is in Fowler's position. As the bone flap is being elevated, the anesthesia care provider states that the patient has become tachycardic and hypotensive, and there has been a sudden drop in oxygen saturation. What is your first action?

> ### "Go To" Activity — Check It Out!
>
> Go to Question #22 under the Perioperative question of the week tab in the Toolbox at http://www.cc-institute.org/toolbox for an additional critical-thinking question.

Activity — Fill in the Blank

The first action in treating laryngospasm is to

_____ .

Activity — Critical Thinking

You are preparing to move a patient to the ICU after surgery to treat a tension pneumothorax following a motor vehicle accident. The patient has a right chest tube in place. How can the patient be safely transported with the chest tube system intact?

Additional Readings/Resources

Girard, N.J. (2012). Silent pain in the neck. *AORN Journal, 95*(2), 312, 266.

Module 4: Fire

OR fires are listed as "sentinel events." An oxygen-rich environment, flammable preps and drapes, and a plethora of ignition sources make the OR an especially high-risk area.

OR fires that involve the airway are some of the most devastating fires that involve patients. Laser and electrosurgical precautions must be implemented to prevent surgical fires of the airway.

Competency Outcomes

To successfully complete the activities in this module, you will need to be able to:

1. Identify steps to minimize the risk of fire.
2. Describe interventions to control a fire in the OR.

Recommended Readings

Alexander's Care of the Patient in Surgery. (2015, 15th ed.), pp. 33-34, 244-246, 640.

Berry and Kohn's Operating Room Technique. (2013, 12th ed.), pp. 224-226.

Perioperative Standards and Recommended Practices. (2014), pp. 126-127, 147-150, 232-236.

Key Words

Burn, explosion, flammable, fuel, ignition source, oxygen, PASS, RACE

Activity — Critical Thinking

Toby, a 28-year-old male, has been admitted to the hospital for elective tonsillectomy/adenoidectomy. He has long hair, which he wears in a pony tail, and a medium length curly beard, trimmed neatly. He is healthy and in good physical shape. He has decided to have this surgery because of the snoring his wife complains about nightly, and the frequent sore throats, which have become annoying. He is a non-smoker. His preoperative assessment reveals nothing remarkable. He takes only occasional ibuprofen or acetaminophen for sore muscles or a headache, a multivitamin, and no prescription meds. He has no known drug allergies. He is 5' 8" and weighs 175 lbs.

Toby is wheeled to the operating room and positioned supine with a foam donut under his head. He is intubated with a cuffed ET tube. The surgery is to be performed with a CO_2 laser and a tonsil tip electrocautery handpiece. The only prep performed is an antiseptic mouthwash swish.

As the surgeon uses the laser for the first time there is a flash of light and suddenly the patient's beard is smoking. Then the surgical drape catches fire!

What are your first actions?

What could you have done to prevent this fire?

Additional Readings/Resources

AORN Fire Safety Toolkit. Retrieved Feb. 15, 2014, from http://www.aorn.org/ Clinical_Practice/ToolKits/Tool_Kits.aspx
Note: Must be an AORN member to access.

Chapp, K., & Lange, L. (2011). Warming blanket head drapes and trapped anesthetic gases: Understanding the fire risk. *AORN Journal, 93*(6), 749-760.

Knudson, L. (2012). Fire safety resources help assess and reduce surgical fire risk. *AORN Journal, 96*(4), C7.

Knudson, L. (2013). Preventing and managing OR fires requires complete team effort. *AORN Journal, 98*(4), C1-C10.

Knudson, L. (2014). In focus: Surgical fire risk reduction strategies. *AORN Journal, 99*(1), C5-C6.

Norton, E., Gorgone, P., & Belanger, B. (2014). Surgical fire risk reduction strategies. *AORN Journal, 99*(1), C5-C6.

Seltzer, J. A. (2010). Flammable prep agents. *AORN Journal, 92*(1), 6.

Steelman, V.M., & Hottel, R.A. (2009). Where there's smoke, there's... . *AORN Journal, 89*(5), 825-827.

Watson, D.S. (2009). Surgical fires: 100% preventable, still a problem. *AORN Journal, 90*(4), 589-593.

Watson, D.S. (2010). New recommendations for prevention of surgical fires. *AORN Journal, 91*(4), 463-469.

"Go To" Activity — Skill Building

Locate the gas shut-off valves, fire extinguishers, and evacuation routes in your department.

Review your facility's policy and procedure related to fire safety. Compare it to AORN's policy and procedure on fire safety in *Perioperative Standards and Recommended Practices*.

Ask your facility's safety officer or local fire department to provide an in-service on fire evacuation methods and use of fire extinguishers.

Participate in fire drills in your facility.

Module 5: Malignant Hyperthermia

Malignant hyperthermia (MH) is a potentially fatal complication of general anesthesia that requires immediate action by the surgical team. Even though it does not occur frequently, the perioperative nurse should be prepared for an MH crisis. Because the condition has a genetic component, all surgical patients should be screened for a family history of MH.

Competency Outcomes

To successfully complete the activities in this module, you will need to be able to:

1. Identify triggering agents that will activate malignant hyperthermia.
2. Recognize signs and symptoms of an impending MH crisis.
3. Describe appropriate nursing interventions when responding to an MH crisis.

Recommended Readings

Alexander's Care of the Patient in Surgery. (2015, 15th ed.), pp. 151-152, 277, 1017.

Berry and Kohn's Operating Room Technique. (2013, 12th ed.), pp. 636-639.

Key Words

Acidosis, calcium, Dantrium, dantrolene sodium, dysrhythmia, hypercarbia, hyperkalemia, hypermetabolic, hyperthermia, tachycardia, trigger

Activity — Do You Know?

Circle the agents known to trigger malignant hyperthermia:

Barbiturates	Ketamine
Benzodiazepines	Lidocaine
Bupivacaine	Morpine sulfate
Dantrolene sodium	Nitrous oxide
Desflurane	Pancuronium
Enflurane	Propofol
Halothane	Sevoflurane
Isoflurane	Succinylcholine

Activity — Critical Thinking

Which of the following is an early sign of malignant hyperthermia?

Elevated temperature   Hyperglycemia   Metabolic acidosis   Tachycardia

---

Case Study Activity

Mr. J. is transported to the OR suite at 0930. He is anesthetized, positioned, prepped, and draped. The surgical checklist is completed, including the time-out, with no issues identified. The surgery begins without incident.

At the same time that the knee prosthesis package is opened and the bone cement delivered to the field and mixed (1100), Mr. J.'s heart rate climbs to 120. The anesthesia care provider notes the patient is requiring more oxygen to maintain a normal oxygen saturation level. The circulating nurse notes that Mr. J.'s skin is becoming mottled with purple splotches. When the anesthesia care provider checks the placement of the endotracheal tube, she notes the jaw muscles are very tight. Mr. J.'s temperature is normal at 36.5° C.

1. Highlight the signs in the scenario indicative of MH.

2. What other conditions might you suspect?

3. What is your first nursing intervention?

Additional Readings/Resources

Hirshey Dirksen, S.J., Van Wicklin, S.A., LeDrut Mashman, D., et al. (2013). Developing effective drills in preparation for a malignant hyperthermia crisis. *AORN Journal, 97*(3), 329-353.

Malignant Hyperthermia Association of the United States (MHAUS). Healthcare professionals home page. Retrieved Feb. 16, 2014, from http://www.mhaus.org/healthcare-professionals/

"Go To" Activity — Check It Out!

Go to Question #7 under the Perioperative question of the week tab in the Toolbox at http://www.cc-institute.org/toolbox for an additional critical-thinking question.

Module 6: Trauma

Trauma care abides by the "golden hour" rule — the time immediately after an injury when interventions are likely to be most successful in achieving optimal outcomes. Nowhere is multidisciplinary collaboration more necessary than in providing care to the critically injured patient.

Competency Outcomes

To successfully complete the activities in this module, you will need to be able to:

1. Anticipate patient's physiologic and emotional response to the mechanism of injury.
2. Select nursing interventions based on prioritization of patient needs.

Recommended Readings

Alexander's Care of the Patient in Surgery. (2015, 15th ed.), Chapter 26: Pediatric surgery (pp. 1065-1069); Chapter 28: Trauma surgery.

Berry and Kohn's Operating Room Technique. (2013, 12th ed.), pp. 85, 126, 513, 575-576, 626-635, 682-683, 733, 744, 765, 800-801, 815-816, 919-920.

Key Words

Acute respiratory distress syndrome, blunt trauma, disseminated intravascular coagulation (DIC), do-not-resuscitate (DNR), end of life care, mechanism of injury, multisystem, organ donor, rapid sequence intubation, trauma

Activity — Critical Thinking

You work in a rural community hospital that provides care to the surrounding ranching community. The hospital has 22 beds, one OR, and a labor deck. Cesarean sections are performed in the main OR. The majority of your surgical population is adults. Two surgeons who are on staff perform general, orthopedic, and gynecologic surgeries. A neurosurgeon, Dr. H., comes in once a month from a major teaching facility and performs lumbar discectomies. An ENT surgeon from the neighboring county's hospital has a weekly schedule of tonsillectomies and myringotomies, which are performed on an outpatient basis. A certified registered nurse anesthetist (CRNA) is the primary anesthesia care provider.

You have completed your schedule for the day, including two lumbar discectomies with Dr. H., when the emergency department (ED) pages you stat. It is 1930 on a Friday evening. When you and Dr. H. arrive, you find the staff busy caring for the victims of a multi-car accident involving three people. The driver of one car managed to walk to a farmhouse to call for help. His injuries include a broken left clavicle and a contusion over his left eye.

The driver of the other car is alert and oriented. Her vital signs are:
> Pulse: 120 bpm
> Respirations: 20/min
> Blood pressure: 96/50 mmHg
> Pulse oximeter: 92% on 2L/O_2
> Temperature: 36.5° C

She is guarding her right abdomen, which is rigid. She has an IV of 0.9% normal saline infusing through a 16 ga intravenous catheter in her right antecubital. A CBC has been sent to the lab. The ED doctor suspects intra-abdominal bleeding.

This patient's primary concern, however, is for her 9-year-old son. He was sleeping in the back seat, not wearing a seat belt, and was ejected from the vehicle. When emergency medical technicians arrived, the child was unresponsive with shallow respirations of 10/minute. He was intubated at the scene. Fluids are being administered through a left tibial intraosseous infusion. Moistened 4X4 sponges have been placed over an open head wound. The child responds with decerebrate posturing to painful stimuli. When Dr. H. removes the sponges, meninges are visible.

The child's vital signs are:
> Pulse: 120 bpm
> Respirations: Ventilated via bag-valve mask at 18 breaths/minute
> Blood pressure: Palpated at 48 mmHg
> Pulse oximeter: 90%
> Temperature: 34.8° C
> Glasgow coma scale: 5

Based on your available resources, discuss your plan of care for these patients.

"Go To" Activity — Check It Out!

Go to Question #12 under the Perioperative question of the week tab in the Toolbox at http://www.cc-institute.org/toolbox for an additional critical-thinking question.

Additional Readings/Resources

Anderson, M., & Leflore, J. (2008). Playing it safe: Simulated team training in the OR. *AORN Journal, 87*(4), 772-779.

Inoue, K. (2010). Caring for the perioperative patient with increased intracranial pressure. *AORN Journal, 91*(4), 511-518.

Neveleff, D.J, Kraiss, L.W., & Schulman, C.S. (2010). Implementing methods to improve perioperative hemostasis in the surgical and trauma settings. *AORN Journal, 92*(5), S1-S15.

Module 7: Disasters

A disaster can be loosely defined as an event that overwhelms available resources. The event will dictate the type of response needed. Perioperative personnel may be mobilized more for their general nursing skills than their perioperative expertise.

Competency Outcomes

To successfully complete the activities in this module, you will need to be able to:

1. Review transmission routes for common bioterrorism agents.
2. Compare The Joint Commission's requirements for emergency preparedness with your facility's disaster plan.

Recommended Readings

Alexander's Care of the Patient in Surgery. (2015, 15th ed.), pp. 84-86.

Berry and Kohn's Operating Room Technique. (2013, 12th ed.), pp. 20-21, 251.

Perioperative Standards and Recommended Practices. (2014), Recommended practices: Prevention of transmissible infections.

Key Words

Bioterroism, bomb, mass casualty, natural disaster, preparedness, terrorism

Activity — Matching

Match the bioterrorism agent to its modes of transmission. Answers may be used more than once.

Anthrax _____

Smallpox _____

Plague _____

Tularemia _____

Botulism _____

A. direct contact　　　E. aerosol

B. indirect contact　　F. infected animal tissue

C. droplet　　　　　　G. contaminated food or water

D. flea or rodent bite　H. arthropod bite

Additional Readings/Resources

Baioni, K., Gneuhs, M., Dickman,L., et al. (2013). Preparing for optimal outcomes: A live evacuation exercise. *AORN Journal, 98*(1), 71-76.

Centers for Disease Control and Prevention. Bioterrorism. Retrieved Feb. 16, 2014, from http://emergency.cdc.gov/bioterrorism/

Centers for Disease Control and Prevention. Emergency preparedness and response: Mass casualty event preparedness and response. Retrieved Feb. 16, 2014, from http://emergency.cdc.gov/masscasualties/

Centers for Disease Control and Prevention. Mass casualties predictor. Retrieved Feb. 16, 2014, from http://www.bt.cdc.gov/masscasualties/predictor.asp

Harrington, S., Gorgone, P., & Jocelyn, J. (2012). Aftermath of an earthquake: A first responder's perspective. *AORN Journal, 96*(4), 419-433.

Knudson, L. (2012). Emergency preparedness helps save lives at University of Colorado Hospital. *AORN Journal, 96*(3), C6-C7.

Knudson, L. (2012). Natural disasters test adaptability of emergency response plans. *AORN Journal, 96*(4), C1-C9.

Knudson, L. (2013). Beth Israel Deaconess coordinates fluid emergency response to Boston bombings. *AORN Journal, 98*(3), C1-C10.

Mitchell, L., Anderle, D., Nastally, K., et al. (2009). Lessons learned from Hurricane Ike. *AORN Journal, 89*(6), 1073-1078.

PBS Nova online (2009). History of biowarfare. Retrieved Feb. 16, 2014, from http://www.pbs.org/wgbh/nova/military/history-biowarfare.html
Note: Available as an interactive video and in print.

Simmons, K., & Adachi, K. (2012). Global collaboration in disaster nursing. *AORN Journal, 96*(2), 196-202.

"Go To" Activity — Check It Out!

Go to Question #50, Emergency situation, under the Perioperative question of the week tab in the Toolbox at http://www.cc-institute.org/toolbox for another critical-thinking activity.

"Go To" Activity — Skill Building

Review your facility's emergency preparedness plan. Are The Joint Commission's requirements for mitigation, preparedness, response, and recovery incorporated?

Offer to update your department's telephone triage list.

Volunteer to serve as a resource for your local Red Cross or community health department.

Chapter Summary

One of the perioperative nurse's most important roles is that of patient advocate. In this role, the nurse must be prepared for any type of emergency that may occur in the surgical practice setting. Teamwork is important in achieving desired outcomes, but it takes on greater significance in an emergency. The perioperative nurse is in the unique role of coordinating the team effort and assisting other team members in appropriately preparing for and responding to an emergency in the OR.

Glossary

Activity — It's Your Turn

Using your resources, define the following terms found in this chapter.

Acidosis —

Acute respiratory distress syndrome (ARDS) —

Allergy —

Anaphylaxis —

Anoxia —

Arterial blood gas —

Aspiration —

Atelectasis —

Bioterrorism —

Bronchospasm —

Cricoid pressure (Sellick manuever) —

Dantrolene sodium (Dantrium) —

Deep vein thrombosis —

Difficult airway —

Disseminated intravascular coagulation (DIC) —

Dysrhythmia —

Embolus —

Hypercarbia —

Hyperkalemia —

Hypoxia —

Laryngospasm —

Latex free —

Latex safe —

PASS —

Pneumothorax —

Pulmonary edema —

Pulmonary embolism —

Pulmonary hypertension —

RACE —

Rapid sequence intubation —

Thrombus —

References

AORN. (2014). *Perioperative Standards and Recommended Practices*. Denver: AORN, Inc.

The Joint Commission. (2014). *Comprehensive Accreditation Manual for Hospitals: The Official Handbook* (Emergency Management). Oakbrook Terrace, IL: The Joint Commission.

Phillips, N. (2013). *Berry and Kohn's Operating Room Technique* (12th ed.). St. Louis: Mosby.

Project Check. Retrieved April 28, 2014, from http://www.projectcheck.org/crisis.html Note: Contains 12 common operating room crises with corresponding checklists. A template is provided to develop a checklist for additional crises.

Rothrock, J.C. (Ed.). (2015). *Alexander's Care of the Patient in Surgery* (15th ed.). St. Louis: Mosby.

U.S. Department of Labor, Occupational Safety and Health Administration (OSHA). Hazard communication. Retrieved Feb. 16, 2014, from http://www.osha.gov/dsg/hazcom/index.html

U.S. Office of Personnel Management (OPM). (1999). Patients' Bill of Rights. Retrieved Feb. 16, 2014, from http://www.opm.gov/healthcare-insurance/healthcare/reference-materials/#url=Bill-of-Rights

Answers to Chapter 7 Activities

Module 1: Anaphylaxis — Pages 211-213

Activity — Critical Thinking

You are assigned to care for Mrs. M., who has been diagnosed with a latex allergy. She is scheduled as the third case of the day. Describe your plan to decrease Mrs. M.'s risk for developing a latex reaction during her perioperative experience.

Responses may vary but should contain the following key components:

1. If possible, move Mrs. M.'s case to the first case of the day, or to another room that has not been used.

2. Identify Mrs. M.'s allergy with a wristband, document on her medical record, and notify other health care providers who will be caring for her.

3. Implement latex precautions. Remove all items containing latex from the room. Post signs indicating "Latex Allergy" on all doors to OR and restrict traffic.

4. If possible, use only latex free items; if not possible, notify surgeon/anesthesia care provider.

5. Have barrier material in room in case latex-containing equipment must be used.

6. Only puncture stoppers of medication vials once.

Source: AORN. (2014). Recommended practices for safe environment of care. In *Perioperative Standards and Recommended Practices*, pp. 241-243. Denver: AORN, Inc.

Activity — Do You Know?

Number the following interventions for a suspected blood transfusion reaction in the appropriate order.

6 - Send a sample of the patient's urine to the lab.
9 - Complete an occurrence/incident report.
1 - Stop the transfusion.
8 - Document and communicate reaction, interventions, and patient responses to next caregiver.
4 - Anticipate orders for emergency drugs.
7 - Monitor the patient carefully.
5 - Return unused blood, tubing, and a sample of the patient's blood to the blood bank.
2 - Replace IV tubing and hang 0.9% sodium chloride.
3 - Report reaction to surgeon and blood bank.

Source: Rothrock, J.C. (Ed.). (2015). *Alexander's Care of the Patient in Surgery* (15th ed., p. 38). St. Louis: Mosby.

Activity — Critical Thinking

Many of the signs and symptoms of a blood transfusion reaction (e.g., chills, backache, shivering) are masked by a general anesthetic. How could you tell if your patient under a general anesthetic is having an adverse reaction to a blood transfusion?

Signs may include blood in the urine, decreased or no urine output, hypotension, hyperthermia, or excessive or unusual bleeding.

Source: Rothrock, J.C. (Ed.). (2015). *Alexander's Care of the Patient in Surgery* (15th ed., p. 38). St. Louis: Mosby.

Module 2: Cardiovascular emergencies — Pages 213-215

Activity — Short Answer

You are monitoring an 83-year-old man who is having a lesion removed from his back under local anesthetic. His pulse and respirations are being assessed manually. He is in the prone position. He complains of shortness of breath, and then chest pain. What actions should be initiated?

Responses may vary but should include the following points:

The surgeon needs to be notified immediately and the surgery terminated. The patient should be returned to a position of comfort in the supine position. Additional assistance should be obtained (e.g., anesthesia care provider, manager, other staff members, the rapid response team, CODE team, 911, etc.). Oxygen should be started per nasal cannula and additional monitoring (blood pressure, EKG, pulse oximeter) should be initiated. An IV line should be started. The CODE or COR cart should be brought to the room. The patient's cardiac history and current medications and allergies should be reviewed.

Source: AORN. (2014). Recommended practices for managing the patient receiving local anesthesia. In *Perioperative Standards and Recommended Practices*, p. 466. Denver: AORN, Inc.

Module 3: Respiratory complications — Pages 215-216

Activity — Critical Thinking

You are the scrub person for a patient scheduled for a craniotomy. The patient is in Fowler's position. As the bone flap is being elevated, the anesthesia care provider announces that the patient has become tachycardic, hypotensive, and there has been a sudden drop in oxygen saturation. What is your first action?

Based on the type of surgery, patient position, and the assessment of the anesthesia care provider, a pulmonary embolism should be suspected. Place bone wax over the exposed bone to seal the vascular bed and prepare to assist the team in placing the patient in Trendelenburg's and inserting a central venous catheter.

Source: Phillips, N. (2013). *Berry and Kohn's Operating Room Technique* (12th ed., pp. 610-611). St. Louis: Mosby.

Activity — Fill in the Blank

The first action in treating laryngospasm is to ***remove the irritating stimulus.***

Source: Rothrock, J.C. (Ed.). (2015). *Alexander's Care of the Patient in Surgery* (15th ed., pp. 274-275). St. Louis: Mosby.

Activity — Critical Thinking

You are preparing to move a patient to ICU after surgery to treat a tension pneumothorax following a motor vehicle accident. The patient has a right chest tube in place. How can the patient be safely transported with the chest tube system intact?

Check that all connections are tight and securely taped.
Ensure dressing on chest around tube is tight and intact.
Monitor patient during transport with pulse ox.
Keep the drainage system lower than patient's chest.
Keep the chest tube as straight as possible; avoid kinks and dependent loops.
Do not clamp the tube unless specifically requested by surgeon.

Sources: Rothrock, J. C. (Ed.). (2015). *Alexander's Care of the Patient in Surgery* (15th ed., p. 877). St. Louis: Mosby. Phillips, N. (2013). *Berry and Kohn's Operating Room Technique* (12th ed., p. 910) St. Louis: Mosby.

Module 4: Fire — Pages 216-218

Activity — Critical Thinking

Toby, a 28-year-old male, has been admitted to the hospital for elective tonsillectomy/adenoidectomy. He has long hair, which he wears in a pony tail, and a medium length curly beard, trimmed neatly. He is healthy and in good physical shape. He has decided to have this surgery because of the snoring his wife complains about nightly, and the frequent sore throats, which have become annoying. He is a non-smoker. His preoperative assessment reveals nothing remarkable. He takes only occasional ibuprofen or acetaminophen for sore muscles or a headache, a multivitamin, and no prescription meds. He has no known drug allergies. He is 5' 8" and weighs 175 lbs.

Toby is wheeled to the operating room and positioned supine with a foam donut under his head. He is intubated with a cuffed ET tube. The surgery is to be performed with a CO_2 laser and a tonsil tip electrocautery handpiece. The only prep performed is an antiseptic mouthwash swish.

As the surgeon uses the laser for the first time there is a flash of light and suddenly the patient's beard is smoking. Then the surgical drape catches fire!

What are your first actions?

- ***Communicate the presence of the fire to all team members.***
- ***Pour saline or water slowly on the patient in the area of the fire.***
- ***Remove the surgical drapes.***

- *Consult with the anesthesia care provider on necessary actions to extinguish an airway fire.*
- *Assist the anesthesia care provider with disconnecting and removing the airway circuit.*
- *Turn off the flow of oxygen.*
- *Remove the ET tube.*
- *Pour saline into the airway if instructed.*
- *Remove any flammable/burning substances from airway.*
- *Re-establish the airway.*
- *Call for help.*
- *Notify the team leader or charge nurse.*
- *Get a fire extinguisher if needed for surrounding area.*

Source: AORN. (2014). Recommended practices for laser safety, p. 150; Recommended practices for safe environment of care, pp. 232-236. In *Perioperative Standards and Recommended Practices*. Denver: AORN, Inc.

What could you have done to prevent this fire?

Coat facial hair with a water based gel and drape Toby with damp towels to further reduce flammability. The ET tube should be laser safe, and the cuff should be filled with saline and dye. Laser instruments (e.g., retractors and suctions) should be non-reflective. ESU handpiece tips should be coated with rubber or a non-reflective material from the manufacturer. Drapes should not be tented to prevent oxygen from collecting under the drape.

Source: AORN. (2014). Recommended practices for laser safety, pp. 144, 147-148; Recommended practices for safe environment of care, pp. 233-234. In *Perioperative Standards and Recommended Practices*. Denver: AORN, Inc.

Module 5: Malignant hyperthermia — Pages 219-221

Activity — Do You Know?

Circle the agents known to trigger malignant hyperthermia:

Desflurane   Enflurane   Halothane   Isoflurane   Sevoflurane   Succinylcholine

Source: Phillips, N. (2013). *Berry and Kohn's Operating Room Technique* (12 ed., p. 636). St. Louis: Mosby.

Activity — Critical Thinking

Which of the following is an early sign of malignant hyperthermia?

Tachycardia

Source: Phillips, N. (2013). *Berry and Kohn's Operating Room Technique* (12 ed., p. 636). St. Louis: Mosby.

Activity — Case Study

Mr. J. is transported to the OR suite at 0930. He is anesthetized, positioned, prepped, and draped. The surgical checklist is completed, including the time-out, with no issues identified. The surgery begins without incident.

At the same time that the knee prosthesis package is opened and the bone cement delivered to the field and mixed (1100), Mr. J.'s heart rate climbs to 120. The anesthesia care provider notes the patient is requiring more oxygen to maintain a normal oxygen saturation level. The circulating nurse notes that Mr. J.'s skin is becoming mottled with purple splotches. When the anesthesia care provider checks the placement of the endotracheal tube, she notes the jaw muscles are very tight. Mr. J.'s temperature is normal at 36.5°C.

1. Highlight the signs in the scenario indicative of MH.

- *He is undergoing general anesthesia.*
- *Mr. J.'s heart rate climbs to 120.*
- *The anesthesia care provider notes the patient is requiring more oxygen to maintain a normal oxygen saturation level.*
- *The circulating nurse notes that Mr. J.'s skin is becoming mottled with purple splotches.*
- *When the anesthesia care provider checks the placement of the endotracheal tube, she notes the jaw muscles are very tight.*

Source: Phillips, N. (2013). *Berry and Kohn's Operating Room Technique* (12 ed., p. 636). St. Louis: Mosby.

2. What other conditions might you suspect?

- *Allergic response to bone cement (methyl methacrylate).*
- *Pulmonary embolism.*
- *Allergic response to drug/anesthetic used intraoperatively.*

3. What is your first nursing intervention?

Assist anesthesia care provider in starting emergency therapy; call for help.

Source: Malignant Hyperthermia Association of the United States. (2014). Managing an MH crisis. Retrieved Feb. 16, 2014, from http://www.mhaus.org/healthcare-professionals/managing-a-crisis

Module 6: Trauma — Pages 221-223

Activity — Critical Thinking

You work in a rural community hospital that provides care to the surrounding ranching community. The hospital has 22 beds, one OR, and a labor deck. Cesarean sections are performed in the main OR. The majority of your surgical population is adults. Two surgeons who are on staff perform general, orthopedic, and gynecologic surgeries. A neurosurgeon, Dr. H., comes in once a month from a major teaching facility and performs lumbar discectomies. An ENT surgeon from the neighboring county's hospital has a weekly schedule of tonsillectomies and myringotomies, which are performed on an outpatient basis. A certified registered nurse anesthetist (CRNA) is the primary anesthesia care provider.

You have completed your schedule for the day, including two lumbar discectomies with Dr. H., when the emergency department (ED) pages you stat. It is 1930 on a Friday evening. When you and Dr. H. arrive, you find the staff busy caring for the victims of a multi-car accident involving three people. The driver of one car managed to walk to a farmhouse to call for help. His injuries include a broken left clavicle and a contusion over his left eye.

The driver of the other car is alert and oriented. Her vital signs are:
>Pulse: 120 bpm
>Respirations: 20/min
>Blood pressure: 96/50 mmHg
>Pulse oximeter: 92% on 2L/O2
>Temperature: 36.5° C

She is guarding her right abdomen, which is rigid. She has an IV of 0.9% normal saline infusing through a 16 ga intravenous catheter in her right antecubital. A CBC has been sent to the lab. The ED doctor suspects intra-abdominal bleeding.

This patient's primary concern, however, is for her 9-year-old son. He was sleeping in the back seat, not wearing a seat belt, and was ejected from the vehicle. When emergency medical technicians arrived, the child was unresponsive with shallow respirations of 10/minute. He was intubated at the scene. Fluids are being administered through a left tibial intraosseous infusion. Moistened 4X4 sponges have been placed over an open head wound. The child responds with decerebrate posturing to painful stimuli. When Dr. H. removes the sponges, meninges are visible.

The child's vital signs are:
>Pulse: 120 bpm
>Respirations: Ventilated via bag-valve mask at 18 breaths/minute
>Blood pressure: Palpated at 48 mmHg
>Pulse oximeter: 90%
>Temperature: 34.8° C
>Glasgow coma scale: 5

Based on your available resources, discuss your plan of care for these patients.

Responses will vary, but should address principles of triage and use of available resources:

This is a difficult situation and there is no one right answer. Resources and patient needs will need to be carefully evaluated.
- ***Two of the three accident victims need immediate surgical interventions. This facility has one operating room.***
- ***The nursing staff's experience is primarily with adults and well children.***
- ***An experienced neurosurgeon is available in-house. A general surgeon is available.***
- ***An anesthesia care provider is available in-house.***
- ***OR staff is available in-house.***

Due to the extensive injuries sustained by the child and the resources available, the health care team may wish to consider transporting him to a level one trauma center and using the hospital OR team to perform an emergency laparotomy for the mother. In any case, additional resources are needed. The hospital's emergency disaster plan should be implemented to procure additional staff.

Source: Rothrock, J.C. (Ed.). (2015). *Alexander's Care of the Patient in Surgery* (15th ed., p. 1066). St. Louis: Mosby.

Module 7: Disasters — Pages 224-225

Activity — Matching

Match the bioterrorism agent to its modes of transmission. Answers may be used more than once.

Anthrax: ***A, C, E***
Smallpox: ***A, B, C, E***
Plague: ***C, D, E***
Tularemia: ***E, F, G, H***
Botulism: ***E, G***

A. direct contact
B. indirect contact
C. droplet
D. flea or rodent bite

E. aerosol
F. infected animal tissue
G. contaminated food or water
H. arthropod bite

Source: Rothrock, J.C. (Ed.). (2015). *Alexander's Care of the Patient in Surgery* (15th ed., pp. 84-86). St. Louis: Mosby.

NOTES

CHAPTER 8:
Management of Personnel, Services, and Materials

> **Test Specifications:**
> *6% of CNOR test questions are based on Management of Personnel, Services, and Materials.*

Introduction

Patient care requires a complex interaction between the perioperative health care team and often highly technologically challenging equipment. It is the perioperative registered nurse's responsibility to ensure that all equipment, supplies, and the necessary expertise to safely care for the patient are assembled in the OR before the procedure begins. The Joint Commission (TJC) (2014) addresses the importance of having all immediate members of the health care team available prior to the beginning of the case as one way to avoid wrong site, wrong procedure, or wrong person surgery. Being prepared not only meets a TJC standard; it demonstrates fiscal responsibility and respect for both the patient's and the health care team's time, and influences patient safety issues such as infection control, pressure ulcers, and anesthetic risks.

This chapter reviews the perioperative nurse's role in the management of personnel, services, and materials and focuses on the following areas:

- The nurse's responsibilities in anticipating, obtaining, and managing the resources needed in operative and invasive procedures.
- Regulatory standards and voluntary guidelines that influence the scope of practice for the interdisciplinary team.
- Factors influencing product evaluation and cost containment.
- The role of health industry representatives and visitors in the perioperative setting.

Module 1: Management of the Interdisciplinary Team

All registered nurses, regardless of specialty, practice under the regulations outlined by their state boards of nursing. The delivery of care is guided by ethical, legal, and moral principles while ensuring privacy, confidentiality, personal dignity, and quality service for each patient. Every nurse must understand these regulations, as well as those from other governmental and regulatory agencies whose standards, policies, guidelines, and recommendations influence safe patient care.

An effective perioperative RN is also an effective manager. The special needs of the patient influence the degree of complexity of the procedure, the number of staff members present, supplies and equipment needed, skill sets required of other members of the health care team, and surgeon practice and preference. Patients and perioperative team members may be put at risk for injury when clinicians use equipment with which they are unfamiliar. Organization, communication, and critical-thinking skills will expedite the safe and timely completion of the procedure and help to ensure optimal patient outcomes. Opportunities for mentoring are practically limitless as the perioperative nurse guides the team in providing safe patient care.

Competency Outcomes

To successfully complete the activities in this module, you will need to be able to:

1. Recognize the responsibility of the perioperative nurse in managing the perioperative environment.
2. Select appropriate tasks to delegate to members of the health care team.
3. Identify the regulations and standards affecting the nurse's practice in the perioperative setting.
4. Demonstrate a commitment to educating/mentoring health care team members.

Recommended Readings

Alexander's Care of the Patient in Surgery. (2015, 15th ed.), Chapter 1: Concepts basic to perioperative nursing.

AORN. Position Statement: Responsibility for mentoring. (Dec. 2009). Position statement: Allied health care providers and support personnel in the perioperative setting. (Feb. 2011). Retrieved Jan. 31, 2014, from http://www.aorn.org/Clinical_Practice/Position_Statements/Position_Statements.aspx.

Berry and Kohn's Operating Room Technique. (2013, 12th ed.), Chapter 1: Perioperative education; Chapter 2: Foundations of perioperative patient care standards; Chapter 4: The perioperative patient care team and credentialing; Chapter 6: Administration of perioperative patient care services.

National Council of State Boards of Nursing. (2014). *Delegation.* Retrieved Jan 31, 2014, from https://www.ncsbn.org/1625.htm

Perioperative Standards and Recommended Practices. (2014):
- Standards of perioperative nursing, pp. 3-17.
- Exhibit B: Perioperative explications for the ANA Code of Ethics for Nurses, pp. 21-42.

- Guidance statement: Perioperative staffing.
- Guidance statement: Safe on-call practices in perioperative practice settings.

Key Words

Allied health care providers, competency, delegation, education, management, patient acuity, scope of practice, support personnel, unlicensed assistive personnel (UAP)

Activity — Do You Know?

1. Circle the following items that cannot be delegated.

Accountability	Task involving independent nursing judgment
Supervision	Making a nursing diagnosis
Responsibility	Providing extensive patient education
Routine task with a predictable outcome	Planning for patient discharge

2. Mark with an "X" all tasks that, according to the National Council of State Boards of Nursing, may be delegated by a perioperative registered nurse.

A. Initial patient assessment to a licensed practical nurse (LPN). _____

B. Standing order for a nursing assistant to insert an indwelling urinary catheter for all patients scheduled for a Cesarean section. ____

C. Changing the rate of oxygen flow for a patient by the transporter.____

D. Application of a tourniquet by a newly hired RNFA whose competency in this task is unknown.____

E. Obtaining informed consent from a surgical patient.____

Activity — Critical Thinking

It is 11:30 on a Friday night. Mr. K., 57 years old, has been admitted to the emergency department of a small community hospital. He has been in a motorcycle accident. His medication history includes warfarin (Coumadin) for atrial fibrillation. He had a large dinner at 7:00 PM.

Diagnostic exams include a computed tomography (CT) scan and x-rays. The CT scan shows bleeding from the spleen. He is cold, clammy, and very pale. His vital signs currently are:

BP: 84/40 mmHg
Respirations: 22 per minute
Pulse: 120 bpm
Temperature: 97.8° F tympanic membrane
Pulse oximeter: 93% on 2 L O_2 per nasal cannula
Pain: 10 on a scale of 0 to 10

His blood pressure is being maintained by rapid infusion of intravenous crystalloids and whole blood while the trauma surgeon and OR team are called in. The OR call team consists of an anesthesia care provider, one RN, one surgical technologist, and one unlicensed assistive personnel. The postanesthesia care unit nurse is typically called in when the surgeon begins closing.

BL is the only perioperative nurse on duty.

1. What options could BL consider in arranging for additional personnel to assist with Mr. K.'s care?

2. What other blood products might BL expect to need for this case?

3. What additional supplies or equipment might be anticipated to be needed in the OR to be prepared for this case?

4. What outside services/resources should be requested?

5. An emergency department RN, SW, has offered to assist anesthesia. What does BL need to do to ensure that this person can safely provide perioperative patient care?

"Go To" Activity — Check It Out!

Go to Question #34, Scope of practice, under the Perioperative question of the week tab in the Toolbox at http://www.cc-institute.org/toolbox for a critical-thinking question.

Additional Readings/ Resources

Hemingway, M., Freehan, M., & Morrissey, L. (2010). Expanding the role of nonclinical personnel in the OR. *AORN Journal, 91*(6), 753-761.

National Council of State Boards of Nursing. (2011, Jan.). NCSBN Model Practice Act and Model Nursing Administrative Rules. Retrieved Feb. 1, 2014, from https://www.ncsbn.org/ Model_Nursing_Practice_Act_ March2011.pdf

---

"Go To" Activity — Skill Building

Look up your state board's rules and regulations governing nursing practice.
    (National Council of State Boards of Nursing [2014]. Boards of Nursing. Retrieved Feb 1, 2014, from https://www.ncsbn.org/boards.htm)

What is your facility's policy on overtime/scheduled call? Compare it to AORN's guidance statement on safe on-call practices.

Review tasks assigned to unlicensed assistive personnel and allied health care providers; compare them to your state board of nursing's statutes on delegation and scope of practice.

Module 2: Principles of Product Evaluation and Cost Containment

The health care facility relies heavily on its nurses' judicious use of supplies and equipment to remain fiscally solvent. Although the OR is considered a revenue generating department, it is also one of the most expensive in terms of capital and supply needs.

The OR plays a large role in contributing to the estimated 6,600 tons of waste generated daily by U.S. health care facilities (AORN, 2014, p. 211). Minimizing waste saves money and allows for more resources to be available for more patients. In a health care environment that reflects cost driven market forces and consumer demand for quality and safety, health care facilities face increasing challenges to implement programs that reduce the amount of waste.

The combination of cost-containment and environmental factors encourages the re-use of supplies whenever safely possible. As end-users, the perioperative RN is in a unique position to recommend the purchase and use of equipment and supplies that are safe, cost-effective, and environmentally friendly. Products selected should promote quality care while discouraging duplication and rapid obsolescence of equipment and supplies.

Competency Outcomes

To successfully complete the activities in this module, you will need to be able to:

1. Identify criteria used in selecting products.
2. Analyze the financial impact of the product on the facility.

3. Promote environmentally conscious initiatives to "go green."

Recommended Readings

Alexander's Care of The Patient in Surgery. (2015, 15th ed.), pp. 102-103.

AORN Position statement. (2009). Environmental responsibility. Retrieved Feb. 1, 2014, from http://www.aorn.org/Clinical_Practice/Position_Statements/Position_Statements. aspx

Berry and Kohn's Operating Room Technique. (2013, 12th ed.), pp. 97, 213, 300-301, 487-488.

Perioperative Standards and Recommended Practices. (2014), Recommended practices:
• Sterilization.
• Product selection in perioperative practice settings.

Key Words

Cost containment, environmental consciousness (go green), fiscal responsibility, product evaluation, product selection, recycling, resource conservation, single-use device (SUD), supply management

---

"Go To" Activity — Check It Out!

Go to Question # 21, Reprocessing single-use items, under the Perioperative question of the week tab in the Toolbox at http://www.cc-institute.org/toolbox for a critical-thinking question related to reprocessing opened but unused sterile items.

Activity — Critical Thinking

Your facility is considering purchasing a new single-use electrosurgical dispersive electrode pad.

1. Who should be on the product evaluation committee?

2. What should be included in the selection criteria for this device?

3. What factors are to be considered in determining the impact of this product on the environment?

4. How can you determine if this product qualifies for reprocessing/reusing?

Additional Readings/Resources

Brusco, J.M., & Ogg, M. Health care waste management and environmentally preferable purchasing. *AORN Journal, 92*(6), S62-S69.

Burlingame, B. (2009). Decreasing the effect of perioperative care on the environment; Starting an OR recycling program. *AORN Journal, 90*(3), 443-446.

Conrardy, J., Hillanbrand, M., Myers, S., & Nussbaum, G.F. (2010). Reducing medical waste. *AORN Journal, 91*(6), 711-721.

Mejia, E., & Sattler, B. (2009). Starting a health care system green team. *AORN Journal, 90*(1), 33-40.

Ogden, J. (2009). Blue wrap recycling: It can be done! *AORN Journal, 89*(4), 739-743.

Pennington, C., & DeRienzo, N.R. (2010). An effective process for making decisions about major operating room purchases. *AORN Journal, 91*(3), 341-349.

Stanton, C. (2011). Selecting products safely. *AORN Journal, 94*(6), S99-S100.

U.S. Food and Drug Administration (FDA). (2013, Dec. 3). Reprocessing of single-use devices. Retrieved Feb.1, 2014, from http://www.fda.gov/MedicalDevices/DeviceRegulationandGuidance/ReprocessingofSingle-UseDevices/default.htm

---

"Go To" Activity — Skill Building

Spend an hour with the material management person from your facility. Review the costs for commonly used equipment and supplies (e.g., instruments, suture, OR furniture). Discuss the process of purchasing supplies and capital equipment.

Volunteer to sit on your facility's product selection committee as a representative from the perioperative department.

Ask personnel who provide instrument repair services for your facility to provide a list of the most frequently damaged instruments. Link care and handling of instruments with repair/replacement costs.

Module 3: Management of Ancillary Personnel in the Perioperative Setting

People who are not typically considered members of the health care team may nevertheless be included in the operative or invasive procedure. As equipment and procedures become more complex, industry specialists frequently assist the perioperative team with products as they are being used. Students from a variety of specialties benefit from exposure to surgery as part of their learning experience. Patient safety, privacy, and confidentiality need to be maintained regardless of the makeup of the health care team.

Competency Outcomes

To successfully complete the activities in this module, you will need to be able to:

1. Manage health care industry representative presence in the procedural setting.
2. Assess appropriateness of visitors in the perioperative area based on patient safety and privacy issues.

Recommended Readings

Alexander's Care of the Patient in Surgery. (2015, 15th ed.), Chapter 1: Concepts basic to perioperative nursing; Chapter 2: Patient safety and risk management.

AORN Position Statement: Allied health care providers and support personnel in the perioperative practice setting. (Feb. 2011). Retrieved Feb. 3, 2014, from http://www. aorn.org/Clinical_Practice/Position_Statements/Position_Statements.aspx

AORN Position Statement: Value of clinical learning activities in the perioperative setting in undergraduate nursing curricula. (Dec. 2009). Retrieved Feb. 3, 2014, from http://www.aorn.org/Clinical_Practice/Position_Statements/Position_Statements.aspx

Berry and Kohn's Operating Room Technique. (2013, 12th ed.), pp. 2-5, 17-18, 42, 51-55, 325-326.

Perioperative Standards and Recommended Practices. (2014).
• Guidance statement: Role of the health care industry representative.
• Recommended practices: Sterilization.
• Recommended practices: Care of instruments.

Key Words

Accountability, ethics, health care industry representative, loaner instrumentation, patient privacy, patient rights, student, vendor, visitor

Case Study Activity, part I

A vendor arrives at your OR at 0715 with a new total knee implant system for Mr. J. that your hospital does not carry. He asks to be present in the OR so that he may better assist the surgeon in placing the implant.

1. What are the issues identified?

2. How would you respond?

Case Study Activity, part II

A student has been assigned to your room to observe Mr. J.'s surgery. What are your responsibilities as:

• an advocate for Mr. J.?

• a preceptor for the student?

"Go To" Activity — Skill Building

Review your facility policy on visitors in OR and compare it to AORN's Recommended Practices on Safe Environment of Care, Recommendations I and II.

Visit your medical staffing office to learn about the privileging process for vendors.

Review your facility's consent form for patient rights related to notification of visitor presence in the OR and right of refusal.

Ask your unit educator to share the syllabus and expected outcomes for student experiences.

Additional Readings/Resources:

Castellucio, D. (2012). Educating for the future. *AORN Journal, 95*(4), 482-491.

DeKastle, R. (2009). Telesurgery: Providing remote surgical observations for students. *AORN Journal, 90*(1), 93-101.

Duro, M. (2011). New IAHCSMM Loaner Instrumentation Position Paper and Policy Template. *AORN Journal, 94*(3), 287-289.

Gregory, S., Bolling, D.R., & Langston, N.F. (2014). Partnerships and new learning models to create the future perioperative nursing workforce. *AORN Journal, 99*(1), 96-105.

Huter-Kunish, G. (2009). Processing loaner instruments in an ambulatory surgery center. *AORN Journal, 89*(5), 861-866. Bonus: Exam questions follow the article.

Martin, K.K. (2011). Meeting the challenge of perioperative education. *AORN Journal, 94*(4), 377-384.

Messina, B.A.M., Ianniciello, J.M., & Escallier, L.A. (2011). Opening the doors to the OR: Providing students with perioperative clinical experiences. *AORN Journal, 94*(2), 180-188.

Mott, J. (2012). Implementation of an intraoperative clinical experience for senior level baccalaureate nursing students. *AORN Journal, 95*(4), 445-452.

Rickets, D.L., & Gray, S. E. (2010). Improving associate degree nursing students' perioperative clinical observation experiences. *AORN Journal, 91*(3), 383-389.

Seavey, R. (2010). Reducing the risks associated with loaner instrumentation and implants. *AORN Journal, 92*(3), 322-331.

> ## "Go To" Activity — Check It Out!
>
> Go to Question # 39, Student placement in the OR, under the Perioperative question of the week tab in the Toolbox at http://www.cc-institute.org/toolbox for a critical-thinking exercise.

Chapter Summary

Effective management of personnel, services, and materials is the cornerstone of assuring the patient a safe and efficient perioperative experience. Following established institutional policies and procedures, professional standards, recommended practices, and guidelines will assist in procuring the resources needed to provide safe care for every patient.

Glossary

Accountability — Being responsible and answerable for actions or inactions of self or others in the context of delegation. Accountability cannot be delegated.

Allied health care provider — Members of health care team distinct from licensed nursing and medical staff. Also known as support personnel.

Code of ethics — Guidelines regarding professional behavior and ethical decision-making. AORN has developed "explications for perioperative nursing" for each statement in the ANA code to provide the context within which perioperative nurses can make ethical decisions.

Competency — Possessing the knowledge and skills necessary to safely perform a task.

Delegation — Transferring to a competent individual the responsibility to perform a selected nursing task in a selected situation. The nurse retains accountability for the delegation. Delegation is limited to situations in which the patient is stable and where the outcome of the delegated task is predictable. It is the responsibility of the delegator to verify competency of the delegatee. Delegation of care is only allowed within the RN scope of practice.

Delegator — The person making the delegation.

Delegatee (also called delegate) — The person receiving the delegation.

Go green — Initiatives to create a culture of environmental responsibility by limiting waste.

Health care industry representative — Health care industry employees who provide services in the perioperative setting including clinical consultants, sales representatives, technicians, and repair/maintenance personnel.

Loaner instrumentation — Borrowed or consigned instruments.

Patient acuity — Categorization of patient's care according to an assessment of his/her nursing care requirements.

Patient rights — Every patient has the right to seek and receive health care provided with respect for his or her self-image and privacy, regardless of race, religion, or culture.

Scope of practice — "Who," "what," "where," "why," and "how" of nursing practice.

Single-use device — A device that has been designed for one use or on one patient during a single procedure.

Supervision — The provision of guidance or direction, evaluation and follow-up by the licensed nurse for accomplishment of a nursing task delegated to unlicensed assistive personnel. Supervision cannot be delegated.

Unlicensed assistive personnel (UAP) — Any unlicensed person, regardless of title, to whom nursing tasks are delegated.

References

American Nurses Association (ANA). (2001). Code of ethics for nurses with interpretive statements. Retrieved Feb. 3, 2014, from http://www.nursingworld.org/codeofethics

AORN. (2014). Exhibit B: Perioperative explications for the ANA Code of Ethics for nurses. In *Perioperative Standards and Recommended Practices*. Denver: AORN, Inc.

AORN. (2014). AORN Guidance statement on role of the health care industry representative. In *Perioperative Standards and Recommended Practices*. Denver: AORN, Inc.

AORN. (2014). AORN Recommended practices for product selection. In *Perioperative Standards and Recommended Practices*. Denver: AORN, Inc.

AORN. (2011, Feb.). Position Statement: Creating a practice environment of safety. Retrieved Feb. 3, 2014, from http://www.aorn.org/Clinical_Practice/Position_Statements/Position_Statements.aspx

AORN. (2009, Dec.) Position statement: Environmental responsibility. Retrieved Feb. 3, 2014, from http://www.aorn.org/Clinical_Practice/Position_Statements/Position_Statements.aspx

The Joint Commission. (2014). National Patient Safety Goals, UP.01.03.01: A time-out is performed before the procedure. Retrieved Jan. 31, 2014, from http://www.joint commission.org/assets/1/6/HAP_NPSG_Chapter_2014.pdf

National Council of State Boards of Nursing. (2013). *Delegation*. Retrieved Feb. 3, 2014, from https://www.ncsbn.org/1625.htm.

Phillips, N. (2013). *Berry and Kohn's Operating Room Technique* (12th ed.). St. Louis: Mosby.

Rothrock, J.C. (Ed.). (2015). *Alexander's Care of the Patient in Surgery* (15th ed.). St. Louis: Mosby.

Answers to Chapter 8 Activities

Module 1: Management of the interdisciplinary team — Pages 237-241

Activity — Do You Know?

1. Circle the following items that cannot be delegated.

Accountability   Task involving independent nursing judgment
Supervision   Making a nursing diagnosis
Responsibility   Providing extensive patient education
Routine task with a   Planning for patient discharge
  predictable outcome

Sources: AORN. (2014). Exhibit B: Perioperative explications for the ANA Code of Ethics for Nurses. In *Perioperative Standards and Recommended Practices*, p. 33; Rothrock, J.C. (Ed.). (2015). *Alexander's Care of the Patient in Surgery* (15th ed.). St. Louis: Mosby, pp. 6-8.

2. Mark with an "X" all tasks that, according to the National Council of State Boards of Nursing, may be delegated by a perioperative registered nurse.

A. Initial patient assessment to a licensed practical nurse (LPN)._____
B. Standing order for a nursing assistant to insert an indwelling urinary catheter in all patients scheduled for a Cesarean section._____
C. Changing the rate of oxygen flow for a patient by the transporter._____
D. Application of a tourniquet by a newly hired RNFA whose competency in this task is unknown._____
E. Obtaining informed consent from a surgical patient._____

Answer: None of the above.

Sources: National Council of State Boards of Nursing. (2013). *Delegation*. Retrieved Feb. 3, 2014, from https://www.ncsbn.org/1625.htm; Rothrock, J.C. (Ed.).(2015). *Alexander's Care of the Patient in Surgery* (15th ed., pp. 42-44). St. Louis: Mosby.

Activity — Critical Thinking

It is 11:30 on a Friday night. Mr. K., 57 years old, has been admitted to the emergency department of a small community hospital. He has been in a motorcycle accident. His medication history includes warfarin (Coumadin) for atrial fibrillation. He had a large dinner at 7:00 PM.

Diagnostic exams include a computed tomography (CT) scan and x-rays. The CT scan shows bleeding from the spleen. He is cold, clammy, and very pale. His vital signs currently are:
   BP: 84/40 mmHg
   Respirations: 22 per minute
   Pulse: 120 bpm
   Temperature: 97.8° F tympanic membrane
   Pulse oximeter: 93% on 2 L O_2 per nasal cannula
   Pain: 10 on a scale of 0 to 10

His blood pressure is being maintained by rapid infusion of intravenous crystalloids and whole blood while the trauma surgeon and OR team are called in. The OR call team consists of an anesthesia care provider, one RN, and one surgical technologist. The postanesthesia care unit nurse is typically called in when the surgeon begins closing.

BL is the only perioperative nurse on duty.

1. What options could BL consider in arranging for additional personnel to assist with Mr. K.'s care?

Responses to Consider:

Because Mr. K. is hemorrhaging severely from his spleen, adequate fluid resuscitation and blood product administration is essential for a positive outcome. BL identifies that he will need additional resources to effectively manage Mr. K. in the OR. Options include:

- *If there is no backup perioperative OR nurse on call, ask the postanesthesia care unit (PACU) RN on call to come in early.*
- *Call the nursing supervisor/house manager for assistance.*
- *If the ED is not too busy, an RN could assist with fluid resuscitation and administration of blood products.*
- *Call the OR manager.*
- *Ask the nursing supervisor/house manager to call other OR staff RNs to come in.*

BL has an opportunity to improve the on-call system for this OR for future emergency cases. By discussing the situation with the surgical services administrator or OR manager and/or offering to lead a team to identify potential solutions and make a recommendation to the administration, a plan can be developed to handle similar situations.

2. What other blood products might BL expect to need for this case?

In addition to fluid volume replacement with IV fluids, the nurse can expect Mr. K. to receive additional plasma expanders and packed cells.

3. What additional supplies or equipment might be anticipated to be needed in the OR to be prepared for this case?

- *Suction should be set up and readily available because Mr. K's recent meal increases the possibililty for vomiting and risk for aspiration. BL should be prepared to assist with a rapid-sequence induction, including cricoid pressure.*

- *Due to severe hemorrhaging from the spleen and the patient's history of anticoagulant use, the following additional supplies and equipment should be available: additional IV fluids, volume expanders, a blood pump, a fluid warmer, blood filters, vascular clamps and suture, an autologous blood transfusion device, a rapid infuser, an arterial line set-up, and extra laparotomy pads and x-ray detectable 4X4 sponges.*

4. What outside services/resources should be requested?

A staff member from the blood bank or the house manager may be able to bring extra units of blood, or bring several units in a cooler. A lab technician could be available to draw blood for arterial blood gases, hemoglobin and hematocrit, and clotting factors. Additional personnel are needed to operate the autologous blood transfusion device and rapid infuser. The trauma surgeon needs an assistant, such as a registered nurse first assistant (RNFA), a physician's assistant (PA), or another physician.

5: An emergency department RN, SW, has offered to assist anesthesia. What does BL need to do to ensure that this person can safely provide perioperative patient care?

Before delegating any tasks, BL should make a reasonable attempt to assess SW's skills and knowledge to safely provide patient care. Equipment, supplies, and resources can vary widely between departments. Answers will vary, but the following should be considered:
- *basic principles of aseptic technique*
- *rapid sequence induction, including Sellick manuever (cricoid pressure)*
- *location of and use of suction apparatus*
- *blood replacement mechanisms, including operation of rapid fluid infuser and fluid warmer*
- *location of emergency supply* cart

Source: AORN. (2014). Exhibit B: Perioperative explications for the ANA Code of Ethics for Nurses, 4.4; Delegation of nursing activities. In *Perioperative Standards and Recommended Practices*, p. 33. Denver: AORN, Inc.

Module 2: Principles of product evaluation and cost containment — Pages 241-243

Activity — Critical Thinking

Your facility is considering purchasing a new single-use electrosurgical dispersive electrode pad.

1. Who should be on the product evaluation committee?

Anyone using the device, educating others on the safe use of the device, or involved with supply procurement/purchasing, including:

- *Staff RNs*
- *Material manager*
- *Financial director*
- *Surgical services administration*
- *Staff development educator*

2. What should be included in the selection criteria for this device?

- *Patient safety*
- *Cost*
- *Compatibility with electrosurgical unit*
- *Warranties/contractual agreements*
- *Procedure-related requirements*
- *Latex free*
- *Ease of use*

3. What factors are to be considered in determining the impact of this product on the environment?

- *Are the product and packaging made of recycled materials?*
- *Can the product be recycled?*
- *What method is used for disposal?*
- *Are packaging and shipping materials kept to a minimum?*

4. How can you determine if this product qualifies for reprocessing/reusing?

When determining if a product labeled as a single-use device should be reprocessed, consider:
- *whether the product is listed on the FDA list of products approved for reprocessing;*
- *the financial effect of the reprocessing program, and*
- *whether the health care organization can accomplish the reprocessing with existing internal or external resources.*

Patient safety should always be the final determining factor. In this case, the danger associated with an electrosurgical adverse event far outweighs any cost benefit associated with reprocessing the electrode pad. A single-use dispersive electrode should be used once and discarded.

Source: AORN. (2014). Recommended Practices: Product selection, pp. 209-211; Electrosurgery, p. 127. In *Perioperative Standards and Recommended Practices*. Denver: AORN, Inc.

Module 3: Management of ancillary personnel in the perioperative setting — Pages 244-246

Activity — Case Study, part I

A vendor arrives at your OR at 0715 with a new total knee implant system for Mr. J. that your hospital does not carry. He asks to be present in the OR so that he may better assist the surgeon in placing the implant.

1. What are the issues identified? *(possible answers)*

- *Patient consent for procedure*
- *Education of team on new system*
- *Credentials/privileges for vendor*
- *Sterilization of implants delivered day of surgery*

2. How would you respond? *(possible answers)*

- *The surgeon must discuss plan for new instrumentation and get consent from patient.*
- *Loaner instrumentation must be processed in accordance with safe sterilization practices; this may necessitate rescheduling case for a later time.*
- *Medical staffing office must be contacted and credentials verified for industry representative.*
- *Staff must be educated on new system.*

Source: AORN. (2014). Guidance statement: The role of the health care industry representative, pp. 603-604; Recommended practices for cleaning and care of surgical instruments and powered equipment, Recommendation III, p. 542. In *Perioperative Standards and Recommended Practices.* Denver: AORN, Inc.

Case Study Activity, part II

A student has been assigned to your room to observe Mr. J.'s surgery. What are your responsibilities as:

(Answers are representative and are not meant to be all-inclusive.)

- an advocate for Mr. J.?

  Ask Mr. J. for his permission to allow the student to observe his surgery.
  Maintain confidentiality of patient documentation.
  Maintain patient privacy during transfer, positioning, and prepping.
  Share and discuss only pertinent information related to Mr. J.'s care.
  Check with unit educator/manager to ensure student has met academic and facility requirements for placement at the facility.

- a preceptor for the student?

  Introduce student to other members of the health care team.
  Facilitate the work environment to make it conducive to learning.
  Model professional behavior.
  Check with unit educator/manager to ensure student has met academic and facility requirements for placement at the facility.
  Obtain objectives and goals for clinical experience and work with student to meet as many as possible.

Sources: AORN. (2014). *Perioperative Standards and Recommended Practices*, Exhibit B: Perioperative explications for the ANA Code of Ethics for Nurses, p. 28. AORN. (Dec. 2009). Position statement: Responsibility for mentoring. Retrieved Feb. 3, 2014, from http://www.aorn.org/Clinical_Practice/Position_Statements/Position_Statements.aspx

NOTES

CHAPTER 9:
Professional Accountability

Test Specifications:
6% of CNOR test questions are based on Professional Accountability.

Introduction

Society holds nurses, individually and collectively, accountable for acting in the public's best interest. Professional accountability, however, goes beyond being an exemplary clinician; a profession is more than a job. A profession includes the expectation of commitment to personal excellence and professional involvement that rises above the expectations of the workplace.

This chapter will help you identify the components of professional responsibility and accountability, and the resources available for functioning effectively as a professional perioperative nurse.

Recommended Reading

Alexander's Care of the Patient in Surgery. (2015, 15th ed.), Chapter 1: Concepts basic to perioperative nursing.

Berry and Kohn's Operating Room Technique. (2013, 12th ed.), Chapter 2: Foundations of perioperative patient care standards; Chapter 6: Administration of perioperative patient services.

Perioperative Standards and Recommended Practices. (2014):
- Standards of perioperative nursing, pp. 3-17.
- Exhibit B: Perioperative explications for the ANA code of ethics for nurses, pp. 21-42.

Module 1: Principles of Social Policy

The nursing profession is defined both legally and by expert practice recommendations. Statutes, regulations, standards, and guidelines that govern the practice of professional nursing are developed by legal entities and experts in the field to protect and promote the welfare of the patients nurses serve. Appendix D provides a list of frequently referenced agencies.

"Scope of practice" relates to WHAT a nurse can do, including what can be delegated and what may not be delegated. "Standards of practice" describe HOW a nurse is expected to practice. Standards describe what experts consider to be the best way to approach clinical challenges to facilitate the best patient outcomes.

"Go To" Activity — Check It Out!
Go to Question # 34, Scope of practice, under the Perioperative question of the week tab in the Toolbox at http://www.cc-institute.org/toolbox for a critical-thinking question.

Competency Outcomes

To successfully complete the activities in this module, you will need to be able to:

1. Examine regulatory agencies' contributions to providing guidance in protecting the patient.
2. Review your state's nurse practice act.
3. Differentiate between scope of practice and standards of practice.

Key Words

Accrediting agency (e.g., TJC, DNV), best practice, board of nursing, community standard, evidence-based practice, guidelines, nurse practice act, position statement, recommended practices, regulation, scope of practice, standard, statute

Additional Readings/Resources

AORN. (2010). State continuing education requirements. *AORN Journal, 92*(6), S120-S122.

Chard, R. (2013). The personal and professional impact of the Future of Nursing report. *AORN Journal, 98*(3), 273-280.

"Go To" Activity — Skill Building
Obtain a copy of the Nurse Practice Act for your state. Compare its scope of practice with your current job description.

Hemingway, M., Freehan, M., & Morrissey, L. (2010). Expanding the role of nonclinical personnel in the OR. *AORN Journal, 91*(6), 753-761.

Activity — Matching

Match the agency with the service it provides (next page).

Association of periOperative Registered Nurses (AORN) _____

Centers for Disease Control and Prevention (CDC) _____

Centers for Medicare and Medicaid Services (CMS) _____

Food and Drug Administration (FDA) _____

Health Information Portability and Accountability Act (HIPAA) _____

Accrediting agencies (e.g., TJC, DNV-GL Healthcare) _____

State board of nursing _____

Surgical Care Improvement Project (SCIP) _____

Occupational Safety and Health Administration (OSHA) _____

> A. Ensures a safe and healthy workplace that would not subject workers to hazards that could result in physical harm or death
>
> B. Identifies preventable conditions and prevents hospitals for billing for these costs
>
> C. Addresses confidentiality of patient information in the medical record and consent processes for access to patients' health information
>
> D. Provides information on infectious diseases
>
> E. Agencies that measure compliance with pre-determined standards, typically through a survey mechanism linked to reimbursement or other financial incentives
>
> F. Combination of governmental/non-governmental organizations focused on improving care by reducing surgical complications
>
> G. Regulates medical devices and pharmaceuticals
>
> H. Professional organization that empowers perioperative nurses with education, networking opportunities, and standards for nursing practice
>
> I. Protects the public's health and welfare by overseeing and ensuring the safe practice of nursing

Module 2: Resources for Professional Growth

Included in the defining characteristics of a professional is the responsibility to evaluate one's own nursing practice in relation to professional practice standards (e.g., AORN's standards and recommended practices) and relevant state and federal regulations. Competency is defined as the application of the "knowledge, skills, and interpersonal abilities in fulfilling functions to provide safe, individualized patient care" (Phillips, 2013, p. 1).

Competency is measured in many different ways, starting with state nursing boards, which validate minimal competency for all nurses to provide safe nursing care. Other methods of assessing competent performance include:

- Direct observation by one's peers or supervisor.
- Audits of patient health care records and other documents.
- Compliance with local, state, and federal regulations.
- Specialty certification.

Competency Outcomes

To successfully complete the activities in this module, you will need to be able to:

1. Define competency.
2. Incorporate best practice standards into professional practice.
3. Identify resources for professional growth.

Key Words

Best practice, competency, competent, continuing education, life long learning, professional organization, self-assessment

---

"Go To" Activity — Scavenger Hunt: AORN Web Site

Locate the following resources on the AORN web site (www.aorn.org):

- Specialty assemblies
- Tool kits
- Position statements
- OR Nurselink
- *AORN Journal*
- Membership benefits

"Go To" Activity — Scavenger Hunt: CCI Web Site

Locate the following resources on the CCI web site (www.cc-institute.org):

- *CNOR Candidate Handbook*
- CCI Study Plan
- Learn about the exam
- Certification webinars:
  - Essentials of CNOR certification
  - An Insider's Look at the CNOR exam
  - CNOR exam: Last minute tips for a painless testing experience

---

"Go To" Activity — Skill Building

Review the competency assessment tools used in your facility. What resources are provided to help you achieve and maintain competence?

Attend an AORN chapter meeting; if already a member, volunteer for a committee or board position.

Organize a study group for other staff members who are preparing for the CNOR exam.

Additional Readings/Resources

AORN. (2010). *Perioperative Competencies, Position Descriptions, and Evaluation tools.* Denver: AORN, Inc.

AORN. (2009). Magnet™ hospitals: The power to attract and retain top OR nurses. *AORN Journal, 90*(4), 609.

Byrne, M., Schroeter, K., & Mower, J. (2010). Perioperative specialty certification: The CNOR as evidence for Magnet™ excellence. *AORN Journal, 91*(5), 618-622.

Gillespie, B.M., & Hamlin, L. (2009). A synthesis of the literature on "competence" as it applies to perioperative nursing. *AORN Journal, 90*(2), 245-258.

Jurkovich, P., Karpiuk, K., & King, C.A. (2010). Magnet™ recognition: Examples of perioperative excellence. *AORN Journal, 91*(2), 292-299.

Stobinski, J.X. (2008). Perioperative nursing competency. *AORN Journal, 88*(3), 417-436.

Sullivan, D., & Stevenson, D. (2009). Promoting professional organization involvement. *AORN Journal, 90*(4), 575-579.

Module 3: Participation in Quality Improvement Activities

The quality improvement process is ingrained in health care systems today and is driven by many national initiatives through reportable quality indicators. Quality improvement projects are often based on best practice recommendations. In turn, the results of these projects can be incorporated into actions to support changes to practice. The success of any quality improvement process hinges on the participation and support of those directly involved in providing patient care, including the nurse who cares for the patient during surgery.

Competency Outcomes

To successfully complete the activities in this module, you will need to be able to:

1. Identify the role of the perioperative nurse in quality improvement.
2. Apply quality improvement principles (e.g., PDSA) in solving perioperative problems.

Key Words

Audit, best practice, change, evidence-based practice, information literacy, measures, performance improvement, Plan-Do-Study-Act, quality assurance, quality improvement, shared governance

Activity — Critical Thinking

During a staff meeting, your director states that surgeons have noted the high quality of nursing care provided to their patients, but they "can never get my 0730 case started on time." Using the Plan-Do-Study-Act method, write the step in the appropriate section for this quality improvement project: :

Plan	**Do**	**Study**	**Act**

_____ Data was collected for 3 months by staff in 0730 cases. An audit tool was completed. The top 5 reasons for a late start were analyzed.

_____ Data showed that most cases were late due to insufficient staff to handle volume of patients in pre-admissions testing for day-of laboratory work.

_____ Steps to address findings include communicating results of audit to appropriate persons/departments.

_____ The objective of this project is to decrease the number of late start 0730 cases. Promoting efficient use of time will allow the following cases to also begin on time, increase patient and surgeon satisfaction, and decrease the amount of overtime for staff. Data will be collected related to late starts, type of case, surgeon, and cause of late start.

"Go To" Activity — Skill Building

Participate in an audit for your department. Offer to help analyze the data and report the results to staff.

Volunteer to sit on the quality improvement committee for your facility.

Submit a comment on an AORN Recommended Practice or Position Statement.

Present a quality improvement or best practice article at your department journal club or in-service.

Additional Readings/Resources

Hanson, D., Hoss, B.L., & Wesorick, B. (2008). Evaluating the evidence: Guidelines. *AORN Journal, 88*(2), 184-196.

Lash, S. (2009). Lean hospitals: Improving quality, patient safety, and employee satisfaction. *AORN Journal, 89*(2), 427-428.

Nakayama, D.K., Bushey, T. N., Hubbard, I., et al. (2010). Using a Plan-Do-Study-Act cycle to introduce a new OR service line. *AORN Journal, 92*(3), 335-343.

Simon, R.W., & Canacari, E. (2012). A practical guide to applying LEAN tools and management principles to health care improvement projects. *AORN Journal, 95*(1), 85-100.

Module 4: Facilitating Professional Behavior

As members of a self-regulated profession, we are accountable to society for our colleagues' practice as well as our own. When disruptive behavior or unsafe practice from any source jeopardizes patient or staff safety, we are obligated to take action.

Competency Outcomes

To successfully complete the activities in this module, you will need to be able to:

1. Choose nursing actions that support patient advocacy.
2. Select behaviors that reflect commitment to professional nursing practice.

Additional Recommended Readings

Alexander's Care of the Patient in Surgery. (2015, 15th ed.), Chapter 3: Workplace issues and staff safety.

AORN. Position statement: Creating a practice environment of safety. (2014). Position statement: Criminalization of human errors in the perioperative setting. (Nov. 2012). Retrieved Jan. 10, 2014, from http://www.aorn.org/Clinical_Practice/Position_Statements/Position_Statements.aspx

Berry and Kohn's Operating Room Technique. (2013, 12th ed.), Section I: Fundamentals of theory and practice.

Key Words

Chain of command, collegiality, ethics, healthy work environment, horizontal violence, just culture, lateral violence, patient advocate, professional standards

Activity — Clinical Scenario

R.S., a certified registered nurse anesthetist, has been practicing as an anesthesia care provider for eight years in the same hospital. R.S. has always been very conscientious in his practice (e.g., conducting thorough preoperative patient interviews, setting up his equipment early, collaborating with all members of the surgical team).

During the past six months, you and other staff members have noticed a change in R.S.'s behavior. He frequently comes to work "just-in-time" and has been late on some occasions. He has become increasingly impatient with patients and coworkers and sometimes appears distracted during longer cases. In addition, the postanesthesia care unit (PACU) nurses are reporting that R.S.'s patients require more pain medication than in the past.

Today, you are assigned to a right hemicolectomy, and R.S. is the anesthesia care provider. Midway through the case, you see R.S. has his head down on the anesthesia machine and appears to be asleep.

1. What actions must be taken?

2. What are your professional and ethical obligations?

"Go To" Activity — Check It Out!

Go to Question #13, Healthy work environment, under the Perioperative question of the week tab in the Toolbox at http://www.cc-institute.org/toolbox for an additional critical-thinking question.

Additional Readings/Resources

Agency for Healthcare Research and Quality (AHRQ). PSNet: Just Culture. Retrieved Feb. 11, 2014, from http://psnet.ahrq.gov/resource.aspx?resourceID=1582
Note: Contains articles, videos, and resources for developing a safe environment for both patients and health care professionals.

AORN. (2007). Human factors toolkit. Retrieved Jan. 10, 2014, from http://www.aorn. org/Clinical_Practice/ToolKits/Tool_Kits.aspx
Note: This resource is for AORN members only.

Bigony, L., Lipke, T.G., Lundberg, A., McGraw, C.A., et al.(2009). Lateral violence in the perioperative setting. *AORN Journal, 89*(4), 688-700.

Chipps, E., Stelmaschuk, S., Albert, N.M., et al. (2013). Workplace bullying in the OR: Results of a descriptive study. *AORN Journal, 98*(5), 479-493.

Costello, J., Clarke, C., Gravely, G., D'Agostino-Rose, et al. (2011). Working together to build a respectful workplace: Transforming OR culture. *AORN Journal, 93*(1), 115-126.

Coursey, J.H., Rodriguez, R.E., Dieckmann, L.S., et al. (2013). Successful implementation of policies addressing lateral violence. *AORN Journal, 97*(1), 101-109.

Dimarino, T.J. (2011). Eliminating lateral violence in the ambulatory setting: One center's strategies. *AORN Journal, 93*(5), 583-588.

Hamlin, L. (2009). The OR and a "just culture." *AORN Journal, 90*(4), 495-498.

Kaplan, K., Mestel, P., & Feldman, D.L. (2010). Creating a culture of mutual respect. *AORN Journal, 91*(4), 495-510.

Kirchner, B. (2009). Safety: Addressing inappropriate behavior in the perioperative workplace. *AORN Journal, 90*(2), 177-180.

McNamara, S. A. (2010). Workplace violence and its effect on patient safety. *AORN Journal, 90*(2), 677-682.

Pashley, H.S. (2010). Changing institutional behaviors and improving patient safety. *AORN Journal, 92*(6), S105-S106.

Rosenstein, A.H. (2010). Measuring and managing the economic impact of disruptive behaviors in the hospital. *Journal of Healthcare Management, 30*(2). DOI: 10.1002/ jhrm.20049. Retrieved Feb. 7, 2014, from http://www.physiciandisruptivebehavior.com/ admin/articles/20.pdf

Chapter Summary

Professionalism in nursing is a personal commitment to patient care based on evidence-based best practices; maintaining currency with changes in the patient population, technology, and the health care environment; and participating actively in the profession through professional organizations. In today's dynamic perioperative environment and diversity of practice settings, the perioperative nurse should continually update and maintain the requisite knowledge and skills as a competent care provider to meet his or her individual professional responsibilities to patients, the profession, and society.

Glossary

Accountability — Being answerable for the consequences/outcomes of one's performance or non-performance of a task, project, or decision for which one is responsible.

Advocacy — Any intervention designed to protect the patient from harm by promoting safe patient care.

Autonomy — In the context of health care, autonomy is the patient's self-determination or ability and power to make his or her own decisions regarding health care.

Beneficence — Doing good; the duty to benefit.

Board of nursing — State governmental agencies that are responsible for the regulation of nursing practice.

Community standard — The practice norm in a specific community, based on resources and the expectations of the consumer.

Competency — The knowledge, skills, and interpersonal abilities needed to fulfill the requirements of the job.

DNV-GL Healthcare — Accrediting body for US hospitals.

Empirical evidence— Information gathered using the five senses.

Ethical practice —- Nursing practice that encompasses ethical principles, follows the ANA Code of Ethics, and meets society's expectations of ethical behavior.

Ethics — Principles of conduct governing an individual or group.

Evidence-based practice — A problem-solving approach to clinical decision making within a health care organization that integrates the best available scientific evidence with the best available experiential (patient and practitioner) evidence; considers internal and external influences on practice; and encourages critical thinking in the judicious application of such evidence to care of the individual patient, patient population, or system (Dearholt & Dang, 2012).

Explication — Explanation.

Horizontal (lateral) violence — Physical assault, threatening behavior, or verbal abuse between co-workers.

Information literacy — The ability to access, evaluate, and ethically use information.

Just culture — An environment that recognizes that even competent personnel make errors. A just culture encourages disclosure of mistakes while maintaining professional accountability.

Nonmaleficence — In the context of health care, acting in a way as to not harm the patient.

Nurse practice act — Regulations outlined by state boards of nursing that define a nurse's scope of practice.

Plan-Do-Study-Act (PDSA) — Standardized process for enabling and evaluating change.

Position statement — Official stand by AORN on current health care issues affecting perioperative nursing practice.

"Professional culture"/culture of professionalism — An environment that encourages and rewards professional behavior, including academic and continuing education, participation in quality improvement and shared governance, involvement in professional organizations, etc.

Quality improvement — Examining processes with the goal of improving them.

Recommended practice — Optimal and achievable perioperative nursing practices as identified by AORN.

Regulation — Rules adopted by administrative agencies (e.g., state boards of nursing) to administer and regulate the profession.

Responsibility — Ownership of a task, project, or assignment.

Scope of practice — Legal delineation of tasks that a nurse can do dependent upon level of education and licensure as determined by the state board of nursing.

Standard of practice — Delineation of best practices based on research evidence and expert opinion, usually targeting specific patient populations.

Statute — Law enacted by the legislature.

References

American Nurses Association (ANA). (2010). *Nursing Scope and Standards of Practice.* Silver Spring, MD: American Nurses Association.

American Nurses Association (ANA). (2010). *Nursing's Social Policy Statement.* Silver Spring, MD: American Nurses Association.

American Nurses Association (ANA). (2001). *Code of Ethics for Nurses with Interpretive Statements*. Silver Spring, MD: American Nurses Association.

AORN. (2014). Exhibit B: Perioperative explications for the ANA Code of Ethics for nurses. In *Perioperative Standards and Recommended Practices*. Denver: AORN, Inc.

AORN. (2014). Standards of perioperative nursing. In *Perioperative Standards and Recommended Practices*. Denver: AORN, Inc.

Dearholt, S.L., & Dang, D. (2012). *The Johns Hopkins Nursing Evidence-based Practice Model and Guidelines*. Baltimore, MD: The Johns Hopkins Hospital & Johns Hopkins University School of Nursing.

Phillips, N. (2013). *Berry and Kohn's Operating Room Technique* (12th ed.). St. Louis: Mosby.

Rothrock, J.C. (Ed.). (2015). *Alexander's Care of the Patient in Surgery* (15th ed.). St. Louis: Mosby.

U.S. Department of Justice, Drug Enforcement Administration, Office of Diversion Control. Drug Addiction in Health Care Professionals. Retrieved Jan. 10, 2014, from http://www.deadiversion.usdoj.gov/pubs/brochures/drug_hc.htm

Answers to Chapter 9 Activities

Module 1: Principles of social policy — Pages 255-257

Activity — Matching

Match the agency with the service it provides (next page):

Association of periOperative Registered Nurses (AORN) - *H*

Centers for Disease Control and Prevention (CDC) - *D*

Centers for Medicare and Medicaid Services (CMS) - *B*

Food and Drug Administration (FDA) - *G*

Health Information Portability and Accountability Act (HIPAA) - *C*

Accrediting agencies (e.g., TJC, DNV-GL Healthcare) - *E*

State board of nursing - *I*

Surgical Care Improvement Project (SCIP) - *F*

Occupational Safety and Health Administration (OSHA) - *A*

A. Ensures a safe and healthy workplace that would not subject workers to hazards that could result in physical harm or death

B. Identifies preventable conditions and prevents hospitals for billing for these costs

C. Addresses confidentiality of patient information in the medical record and consent processes for access to patients' health information

D. Provides information on infectious diseases

E. Agencies that measure compliance with pre-determined standards, typically through a survey mechanism linked to reimbursement or other financial incentives

F. Combination of governmental/non-governmental organizations focused on improving care by reducing surgical complications

G. Regulates medical devices and pharmaceuticals

H. Professional organization that empowers perioperative nurses with education, networking opportunities, and standards for nursing practice

I. Protects the public's health and welfare by overseeing and ensuring the safe practice of nursing

Source: Phillips, N. (2013). *Berry and Kohn's Operating Room Technique,* pp. 18-20. St. Louis: Mosby.

Module 3: Participation in quality improvement activities — Pages 259-261

Activity — Critical Thinking

During a staff meeting, your director states that surgeons have noted the high quality of nursing care provided to their patients, but they "can never get my 0730 case started on time." Using the Plan-Do-Study-Act method, write the step in the appropriate section for this quality improvement project:

           Plan   Do   Study   Act

Do - Data was collected for 3 months by staff in 0730 cases. An audit tool was completed. The top 5 reasons for a late start were analyzed.

Study - Data showed that most cases were late due to insufficient staff to handle volume of patients in pre-admissions testing for day-of laboratory work.

Act - Steps to address findings include communicating results of audit to appropriate persons/departments.

Plan - The objective of this project is to decrease the number of late start 0730 cases. Promoting efficient use of time will allow the following cases to also begin on time, increase patient and surgeon satisfaction, and decrease the amount of overtime for staff. Data will be collected related to late starts, type of case, surgeon, and cause of late start.

Source: Nakayama, D.K., Bushey, T.N., Hubbard, I., et al. (2010). Using a Plan-Do-Study-Act cycle to introduce a new OR service line, pp. 335-336. *AORN Journal, 95*(1).

Module 4: Facilitating professional behavior — Pages 261-263

Activity — Clinical Scenario

R.S., a certified registered nurse anesthetist, has been practicing as an anesthesia care provider for eight years in the same hospital. R.S. has always been very conscientious in his practice (e.g., conducting thorough preoperative patient interviews, setting up his equipment early, collaborating with all members of the surgical team).

During the past six months, you and other staff members have noticed a change in R.S.'s behavior. He frequently comes to work "just-in-time" and has been late on some occasions. He has become increasingly impatient with patients and coworkers and sometimes appears distracted during longer cases. In addition, the postanesthesia care unit (PACU) nurses are reporting that R.S.'s patients require more pain medication than in the past.

Today, you are assigned to a right hemicolectomy, and R.S. is the anesthesia care provider. Midway through the case, you see R.S. has his head down on the anesthesia machine and appears to be asleep.

1. What actions must be taken?

Responses may vary but should contain the following key points:
First and foremost, action must be taken to protect the patient. Notify the charge nurse and the supervising anesthesiologist of the situation so that patient care will not be compromised. Second, you also have an obligation to R.S. to report the situation to his supervisor, so R.S. can be evaluated and receive (or refuse) the appropriate intervention.

2. What are your professional and ethical obligations?

The risk of harm to the patient must be removed. You have a professional and ethical obligation to report your observations immediately to the anesthesiologist supervising R.S. You also should report the situation to your manager following your facility chain of command, because the situation has facility-wide ramifications. The anesthesiologist is responsible for taking action to protect the patient by removing R.S. from the case and replacing him with a capable anesthesia care provider. Perioperative nurses should be aware of various programs and resources available to health care providers affected by mental and physical illness or by personal circumstances (e.g., substance abuse, addiction) that impair their ability to perform the duties of the job.

Source: AORN. (2014). Exhibit B: Perioperative explications for the ANA Code of ethics for nurses. In *Perioperative Standards and Recommended Practices*, pp. 30-31. Denver: AORN, Inc.

APPENDICES

Appendix A: CNOR Exam Study Plan

The Competency & Credentialing Institute often receives requests for information on how to study and what to study when preparing for the CNOR exam. The following information is being offered as an example of how to organize topics and references in developing a study plan. Subjects are arranged by their relationship to commonly encountered perioperative tasks, knowledge, and abilities. The primary general readings cover the broad topic areas of each chapter, and should be read first. The key words can be used to further identify not only what is included in each topic but also act as a reference for individual learning needs. The module-specific readings in the right column are focused on specific areas for additional information.

This tool may be modified for individuals as a self-paced learning aid or used in group settings as part of a CNOR exam prep curriculum. This plan is to be used as a guide only and is not meant to serve as an exhaustive review of all available literature. Information on specific specialties is not included in this plan. Additional methods and resources for studying should be explored based on the needs and experience of the applicant.

Required Reference

*   AORN's *Perioperative Standards and Recommended Practices*, 2014 Edition

Highly Recommended References (either of the following)

*   *Alexander's Care of the Patient in Surgery*, Jane Rothrock, Editor, 15th Edition, Mosby, 2015
*   *Berry and Kohn's Operating Room Technique*, Nancymarie Phillips, Editor, 12th Edition, Mosby, 2013

Additional References

*   *Essentials of Perioperative Nursing*, Spry, C., 5th Edition, 2014
*   *Surgical Technology Principles and Practice,* Fuller, JK., 6th Edition, 2013
*   Pathophysiology Textbook – McCance & Huether and Porth are both very good.
*   Laboratory Manual – Mosby is well regarded, but there are many available.

Key

*   Alexander's – *Alexander's Care of the Patient in Surgery* (2015), 15th Edition
*   S&RP – AORN's *Perioperative Standards and Recommended Practices* (2014); Position statements may be accessed at http://www.aorn.org/PracticeResources/AORNPositionStatements/
*   Berry & Kohn's (B&K) – *Berry and Kohn's Operating Room Technique* (2013), 12th Edition

Chapter 1: Domain 1 — Preoperative patient assessment and diagnosis

Primary General Readings:

- AORN S&RP: Section 1, Standards of perioperative practice; Recommended practices: Medication safety
- *Alexander's Care of the Patient in Surgery*: Chapters 1, 2, 30
- *Berry and Kohn's Operating Room Technique*: Chapters 2, 3, 11, 21

Module	Topics/Key Words	Module-specific Readings
1. Assess the health status of the patient	Age specific, assessment, diagnostic studies, laboratory results, nursing diagnosis, nursing process, patient education, Perioperative Nursing Data Set (PNDS), physical assessment, preoperative fasting	S&RP: Recommended practices: Minimally invasive surgery Information management Alexander's: Unit II, Surgical Interventions B&K: Chapters 7, 8, 9, 25
2. Review of preoperative medications	Allergies, complementary/alternative medicine (CAM), herbs, medication reconciliation, patient/family education, pharmacology, side effects	B&K: Chapter 23 pp. 420-421
3. Initiation of the Universal Protocol	The Joint Commission, preoperative verification, site marking, wrong site, wrong procedure, wrong person	Alexander's: Chapter 20 p. 688
4. Obtaining surgical consent	Alternatives, autonomy, benefits, complications, informed consent, patient rights, privacy, respect, risk	S&RP: Recommended practice: Information management, pp. 448-449
5. Ensuring patient rights/advance directives, DNR	Advance directive, allow natural death (AND), CPR directive, DNR, living will, medical durable power of attorney, Patient Self-Determination Act (PSDA)	S&RP: Position statement: Perioperative care of patients with do-not-resuscitate orders; Perioperative explications 1.4
6. Pain assessment	Analgesia, narcotics, nonpharmacologic interventions, NSAIDS, opioids, pain assessment, pain block, pain intensity scales, PCA, pharmacology, regional anesthesia, self-report, signs, symptoms, The Joint Commission	Alexander's: Chapters 5, 6, 10, 26, 27 B&K: Chapters 8, 30
7. Development of nursing diagnoses	Medical diagnosis, nursing diagnosis, nursing process, PNDS	See Primary General Readings

Chapter 2: Domain 2 — Identify expected outcomes and develop a plan of care

Primary General Readings:

- *Alexander's Care of the Patient in Surgery*: Chapter 1; Unit II: Surgical interventions
- *Berry and Kohn's Operating Room Technique*: Chapters 2, 21, 26

Module	Topics/Key Words	Module-specific Readings
1. Develop measurable patient outcomes from patient assessment data and nursing diagnoses	Measurable, nurse sensitive, nursing intervention, outcome, PNDS	See Primary General Readings
2. Develop an individualized plan of care	Age-specific, nursing diagnoses, nursing interventions, nursing process, patient problems, plan of care	S&RP: Recommended practices for perioperative health care information management, pp. 443-444 B&K: Chapters 7, 9, 11
3. Incorporate patient education into the plan of care	Age-specific, barriers, patient education, teach back	S&RP: Exhibit B, pp. 21-42 Alexander's: Unit III, Special considerations

Chapter 3: Domain 3 — Intraoperative activities

Primary General Readings:

- *Alexander's Care of the Patient in Surgery*: Chapters 2, 4, 6
- *Berry and Kohn's Operating Room Technique*: Chapters 2, 11, 25

Module	Topics/Key Words	Module-specific Readings
1. Introduction of the patient to the operative/procedure area	Behavioral response, beliefs, confidentiality, culture, deep vein thrombosis (DVT), hypothermia, intraoperative, knowledge deficit, patient coping mechanisms, patient education, patient transfer, physiologic response, sequential compression device (SCD), spirituality, stress, time-out, venous stasis	S&RP: Recommended practices: Prevention of unplanned hypothermia Transfer of patient care information Prevention of deep vein thrombosis Guidance Statement: Safe patient handling and movement B&K: Chapters 7, 21
2. Support safe practices regarding anesthesia provider, surgeon, and nurse administered medications	Action, analgesia, anesthetic, cricoid pressure, delivery, documentation, drugs, seven rights, labeling, malignant hyperthermia, medication, medication reconciliation, moderate sedation, patient safety, pharmacology, physical status classification, physiologic response, solutions	S&RP: Recommended practices: Managing the patient receiving moderate sedation/analgesia Medication safety Managing the patient receiving local anesthesia Alexander's: Chapter 5 B&K: Chapters 23, 24

(continued on next page)

Chapter 3: Domain 3 — Intraoperative activities (continued)

Module	Topics/Key Words	Module-specific Readings
3. Incorporate principles of safe positioning	Braden score, Fowler, lateral, lithotomy, nerve injury, positioning, pressure points, prone, reverse Trendelenburg, semi-Fowler, supine, skin integrity, Trendelenburg	S&RP: Recommended practices: Positioning the patient
4. Prepare the surgical site	Antiseptic, cleansing, prep, skin antisepsis, Surgical Care Improvement Project (SCIP), surgical site, wound healing	S&RP: Recommended practices: Preoperative patient skin antisepsis
5. Apply principles of asepsis	Asepsis, gloving, gowning, hand hygiene, sterile field, sterile technique, surgical attire, surgical consciousness, traffic patterns	S&RP: Recommended practices: Surgical attire Hand hygiene Sterile technique Traffic patterns Product selection Prevention of transmissible infections B&K: Chapters 15, 16, 20 pp. 577
6. Provide perioperative nursing care during operative and invasive procedures	Anatomy, hemostasis, implant, invasive procedure, minimally invasive, operation, physiology, specialty, surgery, wound healing	S&RP: Recommended practices: Minimally invasive surgery Surgical tissue banking Alexander's: Chapters 7,8, 9; Unit II, Surgical interventions B&K: Chapters 19, 28, 29, 31, Section 12: Surgical specialties
7. Identify and control environmental factors	Air exchanges, antiseptic, environmental cleaning, humidity, infectious waste, noise, room turnover, spills, temperature, terminal cleaning, traffic patterns, turnover	S&RP: Recommended practices: Environmental cleaning Safe environment of care B&K: Chapters 10, 11, 12, 13
8. Monitor and intervene to reduce the risk of complications and adverse outcomes	Adverse event, body mechanics, chemicals, electrosurgery, ergonomics, equipment testing, fire, laser, National Patient Safety Goals, radiation, patient safety, sharps injury, smoke evacuation	S&RP: Recommended practices: Electrosurgery Laser safety Pneumatic tourniquet Reducing radiological exposure Sharps injury prevention Position statement: Creating a practice environment of safety Alexander's: Chapter 3 B&K: Chapters 13, 20, 22, 27, 31
9. Prepare and label specimens	Culture, documentation, explanted medical device, handling, implanted medical device, specimen, tissue tracking	S&RP: Recommended practices: Care and handling of specimens B&K: Chapter 22

(continued on next page)

Chapter 3: Domain 3 — Intraoperative activities *(continued)*

Module	Topics/Key Words	Module-specific Readings
10. Perform counts	Closing, complication, count, instruments, miscellaneous items, needles, retained item, sharps, sponges	S&RP: Recommended practices: Prevention of retained surgical items Alexander's: Chapter 7
11. Maintain accurate patient records	Confidentiality, documentation, electronic medical record, (EMR), patient record	S&RP: Recommended practices: Information management B&K: Chapters 3, 11

Chapter 4: Domain 4 — Communication

Primary General Readings:
- AORN S&RP: Recommended practices: Transfer of patient care information; Position statement: Creating a practice environment of safety
- *Alexander's Care of the Patient in Surgery*: Chapter 2
- *Berry and Kohn's Operating Room Technique*: Chapters 6, 7, 21

Module	Topics/Key Words	Module-specific Readings
1. Verbal and nonverbal communication	Communication, culture of safety, hand-off, never event, read back, SBAR, standardized communication plan, Universal Protocol, WHO checklist	Alexanders: Chapter 1
2. Written communication	Communication, documentation, HIPAA, National Patient Safety Goals, PNDS, regulatory agency, standardized communication tool, surgical safety checklist, The Joint Commission, WHO checklist	S&RP: Recommended practices: Perioperative health care information management B&K: Chapters 2, 3

Chapter 5: Domain 5 — Transfer of care

Primary General Readings:
- *Berry and Kohn's Operating Room Technique*: Chapters 11, 30

Module	Topics/Key Words	Module-specific Readings
1. Transfer of care among team members	Communication, continuity of care, hand-off, interdisciplinary, transfer of care	S&RP: Recommended practices: Transfer of patient care information Alexander's: Chapter 2; Unit II: Surgical interventions B&K: Chapter 25
2. Discharge planning for the patient leaving the facility	Collaboration, discharge planning, education, health literacy, interdisciplinary, pain management, postoperative plan of care, regulatory guidelines, wound care	Alexander's: Chapters 10, 26, 27

Chapter 6: Domain 6 — Cleaning, disinfecting, packaging, sterilizing, transporting, and storing instruments and supplies

Primary General Readings:

- AORN S&RP: Recommended practices for: Cleaning and care of instruments and powered equipment; Sterilization; Selection and use of packaging systems for sterilization; Cleaning and processing flexible endoscopes
- *Alexander's Care of the Patient in Surgery*: Chapters 4, 8
- *Berry and Kohn's Operating Room Technique*: Chapter 18

Module	Topics/Key Words	Module-specific Readings
1. Microbiological considerations related to infection control principles	Airborne precautions, antisepsis, chain of infection, contact precautions, CJD, CRE, droplet precautions, MDR-TB, MRSA, PPE, standard precautions, transmission-based precautions, VRE	S&RP: Recommended practices: High-level disinfection Prevention of transmissible infections B&K: Chapters 14, 15, 16
2. Cleaning and disinfecting instruments and supplies	AAMI, bioburden, cleaning, critical item, decontamination, disinfection, documentation, enzymatic cleaner, FDA, germicide, high-level disinfection, loaner instrumentation, low-level disinfection, non-critical item, semi-critical item, Spaulding classification	S&RP: Recommended practices: High-level disinfection Guidance statements: Role of the health care industry representative Environmental responsibility B&K: Chapter 17
3. Packaging and sterilization of instruments and supplies	Dynamic air removal, gravity displacement, hydrogen peroxide gas plasma sterilization, immediate use steam sterilization, implants, load, prevacuum, steam, sterilization	See Primary General Readings
4. Principles of transporting and storing sterile supplies	Controlled conditions, event related, shelf life, storage, time related, transportation	See Primary General Readings
5. Principles of biological and chemical monitoring	Biological indicator, Bowie-Dick dynamic air removal test, chemical indicator, emulating indicator, integrating indicator, pressure, process indicator, temperature	See Primary General Readings
6. Safe handling practices for hazardous and biohazardous materials	Anesthesia waste gases, bloodborne pathogen, chemotherapy, hands-free zone, methyl methacrylate, MSDS, neutral zone, sharps safety, smoke plume	S&RP: Recommended practices for safe environment of care Alexander's: Chapter 3 B&K: Chapter 13

Chapter 7: Domain 7 — Emergency situations

Primary General Readings:
- See module-specific readings

Module	Topics/Key Words	Module-specific Readings
1. Anaphylaxis	Allergy, anaphylactic shock, anaphylaxis, latex free, latex safe, sensitivity, transfusion reaction	S&RP: Recommended practices for a safe environment of care Alexander's: pp. 38, 64-65, 113 B&K: pp. 230-231, 248, 632
2. Cardiovascular emergencies	Advanced cardiac life support, autologous blood, blood loss, cardiac arrest, cardiopulmonary resuscitation, circulating blood volume, circulation, deep vein thrombosis, dysrhythmia, embolus, fluid replacement, hemorrhage, hypertension, hypotension, shock, thrombus, transfusion	Alexander's: pp. 231, 275-276, 279-280; Chapters 24, 25 B&K: Chapter 31, pp. 611-624.
3. Respiratory complications	Airway obstruction, anoxia, arterial blood gas, aspiration, atelectasis, bronchospasm, difficult airway, hypoxia, laryngospasm, pneumothorax, pulmonary edema, pulmonary embolism	Alexander's: pp. 140-143, 274-275, 279-280 B&K: Chapter 31, pp. 608-611
4. Fire	Burn, explosion, flammable, fuel, ignition source, oxygen, PASS, RACE	S&RP: pp. 126-127, 147-150, 232-236 Alexander's: pp. 33-34, 244-246, 640 B&K: pp. 224-226
5. Malignant hyperthermia	Acidosis, calcium, Dantrium, dantrolene sodium, dysrhythmia, hypercarbia, hyperkalemia, hypermetabolic, hyperthermia, tachycardia, trigger	Alexander's: pp. 151-152, 277, 1017 B&K: pp. 636-639
6. Trauma	ARDS, blunt trauma, DIC, DNR, end of life care, mechanism of injury, multisystem, organ donor, rapid sequence intubation, trauma	Alexander's: Chapter 26, pp. 1065-1069; Chapter 28 B&K: pp. 85, 126, 513, 575-576, 626-635, 682-683, 733, 744, 765, 800-801, 815-816, 919-920
7. Disasters	Bioterrorism, bomb, mass casualty, natural disaster, preparedness, terrorism	S&RP: Recommended practices: Prevention of transmissible infections Alexander's: pp. 84-86 B&K: pp. 20-21, 251

Chapter 8: Domain 8 — Management of personnel, services, and materials

Primary General Readings:

- *Alexander's Care of the Patient in Surgery*: Chapter 1

Module	Topics/Key Words	Module-specific Readings
1. Management of the interdisciplinary team	Allied health care providers, competency, delegation, staff education, management, patient acuity, scope of practice, support personnel, UAP	S&RP: Position statement: Responsibility for mentoring. Recommended practices: Standards of perioperative nursing, pp. 3-17 Exhibit B, pp. 21-42 Guidance statements: Perioperative staffing; Safe on-call practices B&K: Chapters 1, 2, 4, 6 National Council of State Boards of Nursing, https://www.ncsbn.org/1625.htm
2. Principles of product evaluation and cost containment	Cost containment, environmental consciousness (go green), fiscal responsibility, product evaluation, product selection, recycling, resource conservation, single-use device, supply management	S&RP: Recommended practices: Sterilization Product selection Position statement: Environmental responsibility Alexander's: pp. 102-103 B&K: pp. 97, 213, 300-301
3. Management of ancillary personnel in the perioperative setting	Accountability, ethics, health care industry representative, loaner instrumentation, patient rights, patient privacy, student, vendor, visitor	S&RP: Guidance statement: Role of the health care industry representative Recommended practices: Sterilization Care of instruments Position statement: Allied health care providers and support personnel Value of clinical learning activities in the perioperative setting Alexander's: Chapter 2 B&K: pp. 2-5, 17-18, 42, 51-55, 325-326

Chapter 9: Domain 9 — Professional accountability

Primary General Readings:
- AORN S&RP: Standards, pp. 3-17; Exhibit B, pp. 21-42
- *Alexander's Care of the Patient in Surgery*: Chapter 1
- *Berry and Kohn's Operating Room Technique*: Chapters 2, 4, 6

Module	Topics/Key Words	Module-specific Readings
1. Principles of social policy	Accrediting agency, best practice, board of nursing, community standard, evidence-based practice, guidelines, nurse practice act, position statement, recommended practices, regulation, scope of practice, standard, statute	See Primary General Readings
2. Resources for professional growth	Best practice, competency, continuing education, life long learning, professional organization, self-assessment	See Primary General Readings
3. Participation in quality improvement activities	Audit, best practice, change, evidence-based practice, information literacy, measures, performance improvement, Plan-Do-Study-Act, quality assurance, quality improvement, shared governance	See Primary General Readings
4. Facilitating professional behavior	Chain of command, collegiality, ethics, healthy work environment, horizontal violence, just culture, lateral violence, patient advocate, professional standards	S&RP: Position statements: Creating a practice environment of safety Criminalization of human errors Alexander's: Chapter 3 B&K: Chapters 1, 3, 5

My Personal Study Plan

With the information you found in this *Guide*, use this and the following page to start your own personal study plan. Include timelines, learning needs, additional references and resources, frequently used web sites — anything you need to help organize your schedule and maximize your study time.

My Personal Study Plan, *continued*

Appendix B: Domains for the CNOR Exam

Domain 1 — Preoperative patient assessment and diagnosis

Domain 1: Preoperative Patient Assessment and Diagnosis

Questions on the exam will deal with the following topics:

1. Advance directives and do-not-resuscitate (DNR)
2. Age and culturally appropriate health assessment techniques
3. Anatomy and physiology
4. Approved nursing diagnoses (NANDA International, Inc., *Perioperative Nursing Data Set* [PNDS])
5. Cultural/diversity assessment
6. Diagnostic procedures and results
7. Pain measurement techniques
8. Pathophysiology
9. Pharmacology
10. Universal Protocol
11. Surgical consent

Required Elements of Domain 1

- Confirm patient identity with two patient identifiers, procedure and operative site, side/site marking
- Verify the surgical consent
- Conduct an individualized physical assessment including but not limited to skin integrity and mobility deficits
- Use age and culturally appropriate health assessment and interview techniques
- Collect, analyze, and prioritize patient data (allergies, lab values, other medical conditions, previous relevant surgical history, chart review, NPO status)
- Review medication history (preoperative medications, home medications, alternative and herbal supplements, medical marijuana use, alcohol use, recreational drug use)
- Perform a pain assessment
- Confirm advance directive and DNR status
- Formulate nursing diagnoses
- Document preoperative assessment

Domain 2 — Identify expected outcomes and develop a plan of care

Questions on the exam will deal with the following topics:

1. Age-specific needs
2. Behavioral responses to the operative/invasive experience
3. Communication skills
4. Community and institutional resources

(continued on next page)

5. Disease processes
6. Legal and ethical responsibilities and implications for patient care
7. Nursing process
8. Patient rights and responsibilities
9. Perioperative safety
10. *Perioperative Nursing Data Set* (PNDS)
11. Physiologic responses to the surgical experience
12. Resources for patient/family education
13. Transcultural nursing theory, including cultural and ethnic influences, family patterns, spirituality, and other related practices
14. Teaching/learning needs of patients and families

Required Elements of Domain 2

- Identify potential physiologic responses (e.g., infection, tissue perfusion, thermal regulation) to the operative/invasive experience
- Assess behavioral responses of patient and family (comfort, anxiety, medication, pain management, cultural and spiritual issues) to the operative/invasive procedure
- Incorporate age-specific needs into the plan of care
- Specify diversity needs and requirements (language barriers, attire)
- Perform preoperative teaching
- Collaborate with the multidisciplinary health care team
- Appraise legal and ethical guidelines related to patient care
- Apply principles of perioperative safety (e.g., chemical exposure, radiation, fire, laser, positioning to plan of care)
- Identify and communicate measurable patient outcomes across the continuum of care (hand-offs)

Domain 3 — Intraoperative activities

Questions on the exam will deal with the following topics:
1. Anatomy and physiology
2. Anesthesia management and anesthetic agents
3. Aseptic technique
4. Documentation of all nursing interventions
5. Environmental cleaning (e.g., spills, room turnover, terminal cleaning)
6. Environmental factors (e.g., temperature, humidity, air exchange, noise, traffic patterns)
7. Ergonomics and body mechanics
8. Equipment use per manufacturers' instructions
9. Expected outcomes related to identified interventions
10. Implants and explants (e.g., handling, tracking, sterilization)
11. Intraoperative blood salvage
12. Instruments, supplies, and equipment relating to surgical procedure
13. Medication management, including the seven rights
14. Pain management
15. Patients' rights

(continued on next page)

16. Pharmacology
17. Physiologic responses to the surgical experience
18. Potential complications
19. Preoperative patient preparation activities
20. Prevention of retained surgical items (counts)
21. Principles of infection control
22. Principles of patient/personnel safety
23. Principles of wound healing
24. Problem solving skills
25. Professional standards of care
26. Regulatory guidelines
27. Requirements for handling hazardous materials
28. Requirements for handling specimens
29. Role as a patient advocate
30. Skin antisepsis
31. Smoke plumes
32. Standard and transmission-based precautions
33. Surgical procedure
34. Universal Protocol
35. Wound classification

Required Elements of Domain 3
- Perform Universal Protocol
- Assist with anesthesia management
- Monitor and evaluate the effects of pharmacologic and anesthetic agents
- Label solutions, medications, and medication containers
- Perform proper patient positioning
- Utilize proper body mechanics
- Prepare the surgical site
- Maintain the dignity, modesty, and privacy of the patient
- Select procedure-specific protective barrier materials
- Assess expiration date and package integrity of products
- Maintain a sterile field utilizing aseptic technique
- Perform counts
- Optimize physiologic responses of the patient to the operative/invasive procedure
- Conduct and document intraoperative blood salvage
- Optimize behavioral responses of patient and family (e.g., comfort, anxiety, operative procedure, medication, pain management, cultural, spiritual and ethical issues) to operative/invasive procedure
- Monitor and maintain patient and personnel safety (e.g., chemical, fire, smoke plumes, radiation, laser, positioning)
- Identify and control environmental factors (e.g., noise, temperature, traffic)
- Test and use equipment according to manufacturers' recommendations
- Confirm, prepare, and present implants to sterile field

(continued on next page)

- Prepare explants for final disposition
- Prepare, label, and transport specimens
- Perform or supervise environmental cleaning for room turnover, spills, and terminal cleaning
- Utilize professional standards of care
- Utilize problem-solving skills to facilitate patient care
- Protect patient confidentiality
- Advocate for and protect patients' rights
- Maintain accurate patient records/documentation related to plan of care and nursing interventions

Domain 4 — Communication

Questions on the exam will deal with the following topics:
1. Collaborative reporting to interdisciplinary health care providers (e.g., critical lab values, medical condition, medications, allergies, implants/implantable devices, hand-off, read back verbal orders, communication barriers)
2. Communication techniques
3. Interdisciplinary plan of care
4. Interviewing techniques
5. Medication reconciliation
6. Proper use of documentation tools
7. Regulatory guidelines (e.g., confidentiality)
8. Universal Protocol

Required Elements of Domain 4
- Identify patient barriers to communication and incorporate effective solutions
- Communicate patient status and changes to the interdisciplinary health care providers (e.g., critical lab values, medical condition, medications, allergies, implants/implantable devices)
- Utilize hand-offs and read back for verbal orders
- Maintain patient confidentiality
- Provide information to the patient/family according to HIPAA guidelines (e.g., status, updates)

Domain 5 — Transfer of care

Questions on the exam will deal with the following topics:
1. Coordination of interdisciplinary care services
2. Documentation of the transfer of care
3. Patient postoperative follow-up communication following regulatory guidelines
4. Perioperative patient education techniques
5. Postoperative complications
6. Transfer of care criteria

(continued on next page)

Required Elements of Domain 5
- Evaluate patient status to facilitate transfer to the next level of care (e.g., PACU, ICU, home)
- Collaborate with interdisciplinary services (e.g., nutrition, wound care, social work, visiting nurse, referrals, transportation)
- Document perioperative education
- Document transfer of care
- Provide and document post discharge follow-up communication according to regulatory guidelines

Domain 6 — Cleaning, disinfecting, packaging, sterilizing, transporting, and storing instruments and supplies

Questions on the exam will deal with the following topics:
1. Documentation requirements for sterilization, biological and chemical monitoring
2. Environmental conditions of sterilization and storage areas
3. Handling and disposition of biohazardous materials (e.g., blood, infectious pathogens such as Creutzfeldt-Jakob disease [CJD])
4. Handling and disposition of hazardous materials (e.g., chemotherapy drugs, radioactive materials)
5. Microbiology and infection prevention
6. Regulatory requirements for tracking of materials and instruments brought in from outside the facility
7. Principles of cleaning and disinfection
8. Principles of packaging and sterilizing
9. Principles of transporting and storage
10. Professional and regulatory standards (e.g., AORN Standards and Recommended Practices, Occupational Safety and Health Administration [OSHA], Centers for Disease Control and Prevention [CDC], Association for the Advancement of Medical Instrumentation [AAMI])
11. Standard and transmission-based precautions

Required Elements of Domain 6
- Use appropriate personal protective equipment (PPE)
- Choose the appropriate method for cleaning and disinfection of contaminated equipment and instruments
- Select appropriate packaging
- Determine appropriate sterilization method
- Select appropriate method(s) for biological/chemical monitoring
- Select appropriate methods for transporting and storing processed supplies and instruments
- Monitor environmental conditions (e.g., humidity, temperature) of sterilization and storage areas
- Document actions related to cleaning, disinfecting, packaging, sterilizing, transporting, and storing instruments and supplies

(continued on next page)

- Describe appropriate handling and disposition of hazardous materials (e.g., chemotherapy drugs, radioactive materials)
- Describe appropriate handling and disposition of biohazardous materials (e.g., blood, infectious pathogens such as Creutzfeldt-Jakob disease [CJD])
- Manage materials and instruments brought in from outside the facility

Domain 7 — Emergency situations

Questions on the exam will deal with the following topics:
1. Identification of, preparation for, and nursing interventions related to:
   a. Anaphylaxis
   b. Cardiac arrest
   c. Environmental hazards (e.g., fire)
   d. Malignant hyperthermia (MH)
   e. Natural disasters (e.g., hurricanes, floods, tornados)
   f. Terrorism
   g. Trauma
2. Roles of interdisciplinary health care team members

Required Elements of Domain 7
- Function as a member of the interdisciplinary health care team in the prevention or management of:
  - Anaphylaxis
  - Cardiac arrest
  - Environmental hazards (e.g., fire)
  - Malignant hyperthermia (MH)
  - Natural disasters (e.g., hurricanes, floods, tornados)
  - Terrorism
  - Trauma

Domain 8 — Management of personnel, services, and materials

Questions on the exam will deal with the following topics:
1. Acquiring equipment, supplies, and personnel for proper room preparation
2. Basic management techniques and delegation
3. Environmental consciousness (go green)
4. Principles of product evaluation and cost containment
5. Role of the health care industry representative (HCIR)
6. Role of non-OR personnel (e.g., visitors, students) in the OR
7. Scope of practice

Required Elements of Domain 8
- Utilize critical thinking skills to anticipate the needs for and acquire equipment, supplies, and personnel

(continued on next page)

- Delegate perioperative tasks to appropriate personnel according to regulatory agencies' standards
- Monitor and implement cost-containment measures
- Practice environmental consciousness (go green)
- Supervise, educate, and mentor health care team members
- Manage health care industry representative (HCIR) presence in the OR
- Supervise non-OR personnel, including visitors and students
- Participate in product evaluation/selection

Domain 9 — Professional accountability

Questions on the exam will deal with the following topics:

1. Regulatory standards and voluntary guidelines (e.g., AORN Standards and Recommended Practices, OSHA, ANA Code of Ethics for Nurses with Explications for Perioperative Nurses, state nurse practice act)
2. Scope of practice
3. Resources for professional growth
4. Competence standards in perioperative nursing practice
5. Quality improvement activities for research
6. Quality improvement activities for evidence based practice
7. Quality improvement activities for performance improvement
8. Responsibilities regarding impaired and/or disruptive behavior (patient/family, interdisciplinary health care team members)

Required Elements of Domain 9

- Function within scope of practice
- Demonstrate competence in perioperative nursing practice
- Uphold and act upon ethical and professional standards
- Assess personal limitations and seek assistance as needed
- Identify and utilize resources for professional growth (e.g., shared governance activities, hospital committees, professional organizations)
- Identify quality improvement activities that promote performance improvement, evidence-based practice, and research
- Choose appropriate actions when intervening with impaired/disruptive behavior in patients and/or family members, health care team members

Appendix C: CCI CNOR 2014 Test Specifications

Domains	2014 Final % of items per domain	2014 Final # of items per domain
1. Preoperative Patient Assessment and Diagnosis	14%	26
2. Identify Expected Outcomes and Develop an Individualized Plan of Care	9%	17
3. Intraoperative Activities	31%	57
4. Communication	9%	17
5. Transfer of Care	5%	9
6. Cleaning, Disinfecting, Packaging, Sterilizing, Transporting, and Storing Instruments and Supplies	12%	22
7. Emergency Situations	8%	15
8. Management of Personnel, Services, and Materials	6%	11
9. Professional Accountability	6%	11
TOTAL	*100%*	*185*

Appendix D: Regulatory and Health Care Agencies, Professional Organizations

All website addresses were current as of April 3, 2014.

American Nurses Association (ANA)
http://nursingworld.org/

Association for the Advancement of Medical Instrumentation (AAMI)
http://www.aami.org/

Association of periOperative Registered Nurses (AORN)
http://www.aorn.org

Centers for Disease Control and Prevention (CDC)
http://www.cdc.gov/

Centers for Medicare and Medicaid Services
http://www.cms.gov/

Healthcare Infection Control Practices Advisory Committee (HICPAC)
http://www.cdc.gov/hicpac/index.html

Institute for Healthcare Improvement (IHI)
http://www.ihi.org/

Institutes of Medicine. (Nov., 1999). To Err is Human: Building a Safer Health System.
http://www.napedu/books/0309068371/html/

The Joint Commission
http://www.jointcommission.org/

National Institute for Occupational Safety and Health (NIOSH)
http://www.cdc.gov/niosh/

Surgical Care Improvement Project (SCIP)
http://www.jointcommission.org/surgical_care_improvement_project

U.S. Department of Labor, Occupational Safety and Health Administration (OSHA).
http://www.osha.gov/